PROSTATE CANCER

TOTALLY EXPOSED

&

MY STORY

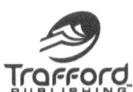

Trafford
PUBLISHING

The information in this book represents an interpretation and views of the facts as seen by the author. It is the personal opinion of the author supported by evidence plus information about the experiences from a patient's perspective. The author is not medically trained nor a fully qualified Health practitioner and is not meant here to replace a GP or medical specialist.

Prostate cancer for many is a distressing condition and for many it is a very personal and private matter. The author has constructed this work as a way of standing with anyone affected by the condition but any suggested action that may be taken as a result of reading this book is only by using the reader's own judgement and assessment of his condition having consulted with a qualified Medical Practitioner.

The author and publisher cannot be held responsible for any action or lack of it taken by a reader who has done so as a result of reading this book.

Any action is taken entirely at the reader's own risk.

The views and experiences expressed in this book are the experience and opinion of the author and any party mentioned may or may not agree with the content.

Order this book online at www.trafford.com/07-1113
or email orders@trafford.com

Most Trafford titles are also available at major online book retailers.

© Copyright 2007 Roger Kenley Dawson.

Note for Librarians: A cataloguing record for this book is available from Library and Archives Canada at www. collectionscanada.ca/amicus/index-e.html

ISBN: 978-1-4251-3061-9

We at Trafford believe that it is the responsibility of us all, as both individuals and corporations, to make choices that are environmentally and socially sound. You, in turn, are supporting this responsible conduct each time you purchase a Trafford book, or make use of our publishing services. To find out how you are helping, please visit www.trafford. com/responsiblepublishing.html

Our mission is to efficiently provide the world's finest, most comprehensive book publishing service, enabling every author to experience success. To find out how to publish your book, your way, and have it available worldwide, visit us online at www. trafford.com/10510

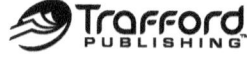

www.trafford.com

North America & international
toll-free: 1 888 232 4444 (USA & Canada)
phone: 250 383 6864 ♦ fax: 250 383 6804
email: info@trafford.com

The United Kingdom & Europe
phone: +44 (0)1865 722 113 ♦ local rate: 0845 230 9601
facsimile: +44 (0)1865 722 868 ♦ email: info.uk@trafford.com

10 9 8 7 6 5 4

INDEX

My intention is for this index to be as user friendly as possible. When sorting the contents to put them in what I thought were orders of importance, it dawned on me that all of the contents are equally important, just in different ways to different people.

In whatever order you read the book, it will make no difference. Unlike Russian dolls, the sections will fit together in the order you choose.

There is some repetition here and there, as some aspects are relevant in different contexts and some things need to be said more than once.

PART ONE

PART TWO

PART THREE

This part describes my experienced from inside as well as outside of my-self and may help some to know what they felt, was also happening inside someone else.

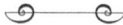

This is how it has changed my outlook on life so far.

   I don't know whether others are affected to this degree but if there is an inclination to seek something else or a different way to be, don't be afraid to move forward.

If anyone wishes to make contact for any reason to do with this book or it's contents, I will be happy to help and the details are in this section.

'You have to expect things of yourselves before you can do them.'
MICHAEL JORDAN

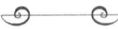

PART ONE

FOREWORD

THE author of this book was diagnosed with prostate cancer in March 2004 and had a radical prostatectomy in June of that year.

Experiencing that plunge into a world of confusion and uncertainty and unable to find the information he needed in order to understand his condition, he formed his mission. This was to do all he could to ensure that as much relevant information as possible regarding prostate cancer would be available in one book to enable the condition to be understood by fellow patients, enabling them to deal more easily with their diagnosis of prostate cancer.

The confusion he felt when sifting through information made what was a bad experience become even worse. Later, on reflection he decided that the often complicated information about prostate cancer could be simplified, making it easier for the patient to understand. Being a layman with regard to medical knowledge, his frustration has motivated the creation of this down to earth plain speaking work and where the few medical terms are used, they are followed by simple explanation.

The author has spoken to many affected men and their families and by doing so has identified the anxieties experienced by patients, both mentally and physically.

An account of his own experience is included and shows how harrowing the diagnosis, treatment and aftermath can be for the patient and his family.

There is full clarification of each step of the way for others, including what questions to ask and what not to accept as a short-straw answer, a perfectly frank attitude is quite evident and literally flows up and out of these pages.

After studying all aspects of prostate cancer through his experience as a patient, as well as investigating expert knowledge, the well-researched information gives all who read this an opportunity to view their condition with optimism. He believes that a better understanding of their condition, why it is there and what can be done about it, will give any man (and his family) a more positive outlook and reinforce their ability to claim his future.

This book has the unique quality of being written by someone who has lived through and is still living through the very personal experience of prostate cancer. His desire to share his experience and his optimism in coming to terms with this challenging condition is clear.

There are no punches pulled in pointing to where the damage we endure each day to our body is coming from.

It is written in everyday language for all who understand English.

Captured here is the positive approach to accepting, dealing with and overcoming the negative effects of this condition.

Anyone reading this who is affected by prostate cancer cannot help but to be encouraged to a new way or level of thinking by the straight talking, honest delivery.

The text is jargon free, no gobbledygook or padding, just straight talking about a serious subject.

THANKS

'Those that fail to learn from history, are doomed to repeat it.'
WINSTON CHURCHILL.

I GIVE my heartfelt thanks to every person who has played a part in my life since the beginning of March 2004.

Dr Pathak. MBE. My GP whose straight manner and keen sense of purpose, picked up with minimal information from me, sufficient to establish the need for me to have a blood test to discover PSA (see PSA chapter) levels.

The staff at the Nottingham City Hospital Urology Department were faultless in their caring and consideration for me while I was undergoing treatment as an inpatient.

My particular thanks go to a skilled and justifiably confident

Mr. Owen Cole and his team whose sincerity and sense of purpose is unquestionably commendable. To Nick and Jane and their colleagues who monitored my recovery after the operation and Elly who still keeps in touch with me from time to time to ask that I am alright. I thank also all of the others involved whose names I don't remember, while the memory of their commitment and sense of task never leaves me.

The team of district nurses who attended me after leaving hospital brought with them a reassurance and professionalism that can only really be appreciated when you have had experience of their attention.

I know that people are paid for what they do but it is important if not only for our own good, to appreciate the attitude and skills of all those people who work in the NHS who improve the quality as well as increasing the length of our lives whenever it is possible.

My beautiful wife who has stayed positive for me throughout this life changing experience is a soul mate without a doubt. The very dark days that have been and gone have at times been chasms to the core of my being; without Vicky calling me across the voids, I don't know where I might be today.

Daughter Bev, sons, Richard, Wayne and Gareth along with Janet, my sister and my dear mother as well as our extended family in every direction are all strong and God sent people and I love them all.

Our personal friends Martin and Pat Woodland very kindly gave me accommodation after my operation so that I could be nearer to the hospital where I was being treated than I otherwise would have been. I thank them for their kindness and much appreciate their good nature.

The list is too long to mention here of the goodwill messages I received from all of my friends and colleagues. I have personally thanked every one of them.

Roger Kenley Dawson

'Be who you are and say what you feel because those who
mind don't matter and those who matter don't mind.'
DR SEUSS.

AUTHOR

'Experience is not what happens to a man.
It is what a man does with what happens to him.'
ALDOUS HUXLEY

Hello,

My name is Roger Kenley Dawson. Although I don't know you at this time, if you have had a diagnosis of prostate cancer, I believe I have a good idea how you may be feeling.

I was knocked off my feet when diagnosed with prostate cancer (PC) and over the course of a few days as I was reconstituting my senses, my outlook on life changed. It doesn't hit everyone in exactly the same way but the chances are that you and I have a lot in common.

If you have been looking for information about PC as I was and can't find it written in a way that you can understand and put it all together in your head then keep reading. I looked all over and couldn't find a book written in a way I could fully understand or that gave me only information that was relevant to me personally.

Pages overflowing with information, most of which didn't matter to me was not what I was looking for. I wanted just to understand what prostate cancer was and what was happening inside of me.

Feeling frustrated, I remember thinking that instead of being misled by stuff on the internet and confused by books full of medical terminology, it would be really good if there was one book written by someone who had gone through the experience, which would give a general understanding about the disease and what to expect in the future, in language I could understand. I couldn't find a book like that so I decided to write one. At the very least it would fill the gap I had discovered, for those who would be in my shoes later on.

Whether you are new to a prostate cancer condition and struggling to understand what is happening to you, or you have been living with it and have a nagging feeling that you could be doing more for yourself but you are not sure how or what, you may find this book very useful.

My intention is to relay my thoughts and experiences as well as that of others to you so that you can understand we are all affected pretty much in the same way from initial diagnosis, albeit in varying degrees, through the various stages of mental anguish and subsequent treatment.

When you have reached a point where you understand what is happening to you and the mystery is out of the way, it is easier to be more progressive about what you can do about your future health and well-being.

Understanding the condition and how it affects us is a good place to start a path to a better way to be, both physically and mentally.

By looking at the proliferation of PC in the general population, we will come to understand that as individuals we are far from alone with this problem, so let us absorb the facts of the wider picture first and the numbers affected, then move on to concentrate on the individual.

PC is the fastest growing physical health problem in men in the Western world and is responsible for more deaths than just about any other specific disease. Deaths from PC are often recorded as having been caused by other types of cancer such as lung cancer, when in reality the cause is prostate cancer, which has spread to a secondary position. This distorts the reality of the numbers of deaths, which if the truth were known is much higher than statistics show.

For a start, the extent of the problem of PC in the UK goes like this; a cancer will affect one in three males at some time in their life. Current figures illustrate that one in eleven men will be affected by prostate cancer from the age of fifty. From this we know that 1 in every 3.6, or 28% of all cancers in men will be PC, a staggering amount with numbers not far behind cases of breast cancer in women.

These are National statistics and give the broad-brush picture of the problem. When we look at the position from the point of view of the individual, our immediate family history becomes more relevant. Not only have we a greater than 1 in 11 chance of developing the condition but if father had or has prostate cancer then the chance of son developing the condition increases to one in six. Two close blood relatives having the condition increase the likelihood of son getting it to one in three. This is not a rule of thumb but is correct information drawn from statistics gathered so far.

Close female relatives who have breast cancer also have a bearing on the potential of PC affecting a male offspring or sibling. Composite figures are not available but it is known that PC is more likely to occur in families without history of PC but occurrence of breast cancer, than it is in families without history of PC and no occurrence of breast cancer. Being aware of these facts helps, as anyone in the position of having close relatives with the condition is alerted to monitor his prostate health more closely than he may otherwise need to.

The odds for generating the condition are greater still should you happen to be of African or Caribbean descent. The condition tends to be more aggressive in black skinned people and for some reason the cancer is discovered later in its progress in black skinned people, as a consequence a higher percentage of men with black skin who have prostate cancer, die from it.

Men whose origins are Asian are much less prone to developing the condition. The reasons for these differences are not known as yet and although much headway is being made in the treatment and management of this condition, according to those better placed to know, there is as yet no indication for a sensible answer.

When immigrants from the East adopt Western lifestyles, they too begin to be affected with many diseases of the Western world, so be assured it is the way we live and not a fault in our personal construction that causes cancers. Prostate cancer is not hereditary, ever.

The previous information may not make any difference to our individual condition but it does enable us to put things into perspective. We should now have a more balanced view and realise that we are by no means on our own with this encounter nor have we been singled out for merciless revenge for something we have done wrong in the past.

What is happening is we are entering what for us is new territory, but where so many others are already, and untold numbers have been before.

Any new territory even one we have chosen, say moving house or job, inevitably brings apprehensions and concerns. These decline when we start to find our way about, and decline more quickly when we understand and choose to accept the changes.

Knowing how I have been affected by this intrusion and speaking to many more affected by the same thing has made me aware that fundamentally we are all similar in our responses to illness. From that awareness came the desire to reach out to those who do not have the opportunity or inclination to speak about their feelings with regard to their condition. I now know they are further damaged by their decision to suffer in silence.

Shame and guilt affect so many who feel responsible for their condition along with the feeling of letting down those around them.

Prostate cancer affects men and their families in various ways both bodily and emotionally. Low-grade (slow growing) cancers may have little or no effect on the person and those with low-grade cancers may continue to live their lives to the full term without symptoms. In others, cancers are more aggressive, presenting symptoms, and in some cases do shorten life expectancy. Men react differently to the change in their circumstances according to how they see life but the sometimes unpredictable aspects and varying symptoms of PC do cause distress and confusion to those affected.

I may be a bit self indulgent in some parts of this book but from the start, the intention has been to give a positive response to the negative inner effects of being told you have an aggressive cancer. Being human, the intention isn't always followed through though, is it.

If I can be self indulgent, then so can you. There may be times when you want to feel sorry for yourself or out of frustration from symptoms, shed a few tears, that is ok. Just recognise that you are having a bout of self-pity, give yourself permission to have a bout of self-pity, accept it and let it pass. Don't punish yourself for feeling overwhelmed at times, it will make you feel even worse.

The population is affected in terms of percentages and lifestyles when PC is being studied on a national scale. It is a different world when giving consideration to the way individuals are affected, whatever their age, colour or background, when diagnosed with the condition.

Since being diagnosed with PC the sheer shock of it all, diagnosis, treatment and aftermath has changed the way I look at life completely. I go for the periodic check-ups and will continue to do so but my life consists of every second of every day.

I am now 59 years old, fit and cheerful. I eat well and I look forward to getting up in the morning…every morning. On top of all that I have discovered things I never knew existed. Time and life have become precious to me.

It hasn't been quite like that all of the time though, when first diagnosed despondency and dark clouds were all around, much the same feelings that affect almost everyone else when their condition is first detected.

Living a busy life, paying little attention to yourself is all very well while things are ok, then the sudden realisation that life, particularly your own life is finite brings a profound effect on most of us and I am included in that number.

As a person I began to change. Suddenly I was living in the moment in my head, rather than seeing the bigger picture view of things that had mostly been the way I looked at life previously. My focus changed to our future and me.

The only way I could see myself dealing with this new situation was to find as much information as possible about it, from wherever I could. This need to comprehend what was happening to me was the beginning of a process that helped me to start to tackle it from inside myself, as well as from the outside.

I set about becoming an expert on the subject. I don't know whether it was logic or intuition but something told me that there must be a cure or counter process for everything that appears on the globe, it just needs finding.

Desire with urgency created the initial surge of enquiring and reading, then thinking further, I became conscious of the fact that there are hundreds of people spending their professional lives searching for these answers; perhaps I wasn't best placed to find the solution. On the other hand I thought, maybe I could come up with something as I had no medical or scientific training and I think we all know that having no knowledge of something can sometimes give a clear view as no mental filters have been installed.

First I scoured the Internet and reference areas in the local library, then on to 'Ottakars' and 'Waterstones' the book retailers along with 'W.H.

Smiths' and the like looking for good sound information on the subject. A collection of reading matter soon accumulated, the contents of which I hoped would lead me to a formula to beat this unwelcome intruder. Somewhere in all of this was the answer or part of the answer I was looking for.

The next period of my life I was to research, and study, and enquire, and feel sorry for myself, and pray, and become stronger, and find the conviction that I was going to beat this, with the help of others of course.

As you are reading this book, it is more than likely that your life, or someone who is close to you, has been touched by, interfered with or turned completely upside down just as mine was, or ours was, with a similar diagnosis. Make no mistake about this, I have absolute empathy with you whether diagnosed yourself or you are searching to help a loved one with a diagnosis. Take heart from the fact that now you know that every day is a miracle of life and if previously you may have squandered some of those days, you have been given the opportunity to discover how precious this time is for all of us.

The majority of the information I came across when first searching, seemed to me to be either very complicated and inconsistent, sausage machine material, contradictory or not relevant to me.

Some of it was very specific, only to be followed by little advice or suggestion as to how to move forward from that point. Not very joined up information.

Alternative information gave many recommendations for strict diet and lifestyle changes. I wouldn't say that coping with all of the recommended changes was unachievable but attempting to make the changes added to the stress levels and this led to heavy feelings of confusion and at times depression would set in due to frustration.

Trying to do the best for yourself is at least a challenge and at worst impossible, when you are not well and becoming bewildered with conflicting information.

The endless medical details and micro-sciences coupled with theories as to what does and doesn't cause PC creates a fog-like environment and hampers the search for the truth. My thoughts were that something has caused this to happen, if it can be caused to happen it can be caused to go away.

I sorted out the information that I felt was important to know about, both before and after diagnosis, and it is here.

Studying foodstuffs that have taken the blame for causing cancers for instance was difficult as we live in a world of conspiracies and ineptitude where information about things we use, drink and eat is not readily available.

Over the last twenty-five years or so all manner of things have been blamed, with huge press headlines, for causing cancers. Everyday foodstuff such as sugar, potato crisps, dairy produce, in fact most food items have been pointed to at one time or another as having cancer-causing properties.

We maintain out bodies by eating and drinking and it has to be accepted that some things we take in do cause illness to develop. When we know of these things, we can choose to continue to have them or choose not to. It is those things we are not informed about that are known to overload our immune system, that probably contribute much more to illness by undermining our natural ability to protect our health.

High on the list of 'BEWARE' factors are items that for years have been known to definitely create changes in the human body that the body itself does not know how to deal with. One of these items is sold in major shop chains all over the UK without any warning of the anti-life properties it creates.

Microwave ovens, sold in the UK with no regard to radiation health warnings are killers, banned from sale in the Soviet Union in 1976 on public health grounds.

Fluoride, which is in toothpastes that we buy, has no health warning attached and is a killer. It is even added to the water we drink from our taps at home even though it is known to cause bone cancer in young males.

More on these things later.

I find it extremely annoying that the best of information is not made available to enable us to make up our own minds regarding our own welfare. If the truth as is known was made more readily accessible and public welfare was a higher priority than profit, we could all choose to be more responsible to and for ourselves in many ways.

At the present time we have lived the way we have learned to live and arrived at a place where we are being told we have cancer. It is no good wishing we had done things differently because the past has gone, but we can decide to do things differently in the future. For now though what matters is, what is it that is wrong with me, what can be done, what if any are the complications and unfolding events likely to be.

After reading this book, if there is some particular aspect you would like to discuss, details are in the back as to how you can contact me.

Please bear in mind that I am a fellow patient, and although an extremely knowledgeable one these days prepared to help wherever possible, I am not instead of your GP or specialist.

I ask that in order for you to start to feel better about yourself, read what I have to say about prostate cancer, how it affected me, how it has affected others I have spoken to and think how similarly or not it affects you. Arriving at a point where you know you are among many others sharing similar experience will if you let it, allow some of the anxiety to subside. Then we can move on with positive steps.

You will be amazed at how many men you know, are going through the same experience. They may not have said anything to you but then, you know what men are like for speaking about their problems, particularly personal problems and more particularly below the belt personal problems.

Try telling one or two colleagues that you have the condition and see how many respond with knowledge of others they know, or members of their own family who are in the same position.

CAUTION. Be aware that there are plenty of people in the world waiting to take money from you as payment for promised cures. The real downside of falling for a quack remedy is that when we find that they don't work we can easily become disillusioned. It can also work to undermine our willingness to try other things. Worst still, when something we put our trust in proves to be useless, it can serve to make us lose faith in our own judgement and if we are at a low ebb, lose faith in ourselves. This can further undermine our immune system.

The Internet has umpteen sites containing promises of quick cures that can charm even the most discerning amongst us into parting with our hard earned cash. I am not qualified to say whether or not these remedies work, but I do think that if they did work we would be seeing them in every chemist shop on the High Street and PC would be a thing of the past.

It is difficult to know what is genuine and what isn't, just be sensible about it and talk to other people who may feel they have been helped with anything that you feel drawn towards. If there are no endorsements from real people you can speak to, then you may choose to turn away from that particular offered item.

If the remarkable cures have helped 'Mr. S from Sevenoaks' or 'Brian from Stourbridge' you might want to think twice before parting with your valuable resource.

Sometimes we can be our own worst enemy, particularly when we want instant solutions to health problems.

It can be the same with accounts from others regarding illness. Listening to second hand information that might be correct for someone else but no good at all for you provides only confusion and uses up priceless nervous energy. Gather information, yes, then make sure that you are comparing like for like before making any judgment.

Everything that you have ever done at any time, whether right or wrong, good or bad, has started off from one point and that single one point is your 'intention'. Without intention you wouldn't get out of bed in the morning.

What is your intention right now with regard to your condition? Is it to work at getting topside of it or is it to say 'well, if it was meant to be, it will be'. The choice you make will determine your attitude from now into your future and your attitude will have a bearing on all of your health.

Read, understand, change your mind and claim your future.

Everything I have written here has been with you in mind, so this is for you, read it, understand it, know it is right and live your life.

AN OVERVIEW

'An optimist is a pessimist with full knowledge of the facts'
ROGER KENLEY DAWSON

WITNESSING the confusion that engulfs men who are diagnosed with prostate cancer inspired me to gather information from them in order to understand the effects of PC as much as possible. I have tapped into what seemed to be confusing issues and set out to explain them. Knowing that this particular illness is on the increase and most of those destined to become affected are past fifty and apparently, don't tend to read very much these days, I have kept things simple and to the point.

I am living with the outcome of a 'radical prostatectomy', which is the complete removal of the prostate gland and a degree of surrounding tissue. The medical experiences and processes I have been exposed to were totally new to me as was the strange language being used, all the more strange as it was being used to describe what was happening, and continues to happen to me.

When suddenly launched into an hospital environment the onslaught of attention can be overwhelming at times, not least so because of the other times when nothing seems to be happening. Many people from all sorts of backgrounds with a variety of reasons for being in the same place as me emerged then disappeared.

At times I actually felt like an intruder, that my illness was separate to me and I, the me in all of this, just happened to be there. It really is an awakener when you are not familiar, to see how many people become involved in health processes in hospitals.

For me, it was Surgeon, Radiographers, Registrars, Nurses with varying duties, Advisory staff, Laboratory Personnel, Administration staff and a raft of other people whose purpose for being involved, I am not really sure of.

Well, I hadn't seen much of the inside of hospitals for years so it was likely to be a shock anyway.

What did happen though was, I started to notice what I was noticing, which may sound strange only, as my lifetime experience of taking an objective view of all that generally happens around me dropped into gear, I became alert to the effects the hospital experience was having on other people.

It soon became apparent that many other men who were there as patients were being affected in many different ways, their body language and facial expressions revealed a mixture of states of mind.

It was at the earlier visits I made to the hospital that I realised just how many people are having treatment and how much they are affected by it. The sheer numbers of people attending the hospital showed me how big an industry healthcare is. It soon became clear that the workload on staff made it seem impossible for patients to get the time they felt the need for, with their respective staff members.

So much difference can be made to a person's life just by taking time and being interested in that person, particularly at a time of illness.

Putting yourself mentally into the position of another before attempting to understand why they act in the way they do is a settling, calming and helpful exercise.

For most people, if we are willing to give it a try, giving time to people who are suffering with debilitating illness can actually make us feel better. Are you one of those people? Don't dismiss the idea, give it some thought. It is a win-win scenario. If you find that your condition is getting you down because you are sitting thinking about it, go and listen to someone else's troubles, it will take you out of yourself for a while, good therapy.

During my time in hospital, I was surprised at the level of commitment from all concerned. Having constantly read in the press how bad the NHS is, I wasn't sure what to expect really but as it turned out, I was given all I needed to get me through what was physically and mentally for me, a bad time.

For those in-patients who were short of visitors for whatever reason, the hospital was a lonely place, even though there was no shortage of people around. The emotional effect on some was obvious, but being a realist, I know it is unreasonable to expect those dedicated to providing all things necessary on a practical level to add further time and empathy to anything more than the tasks to hand. Their nervous energy would soon be depleted and in the long run it would be counter productive.

The psychological canyon between doctors and patients was shouting for a bridge but no one would hear. Apart from the opposing positions of each, the worldly, well-informed and focused surgeons were half a world away from the less knowledgeable older generation of patients, most of whose awareness of their internal mechanisms stopped just short of knowing how they managed to get fluff in their belly button.

I say this to emphasise the difficult situation that exists. The ideal would be to have a liaison person to serve as interpreter for the patient.

Being informed that I had a cancer shook me to the roots, awakening sensitivities and abilities in me that I never knew were there, well perhaps I did know but didn't pay attention to them in the way that I should have. I certainly pay attention to them now.

What might you do about your potential?

How is your thinking different from before?

Do you feel that there is so much you want to do and all of a sudden time is taking a faster pace?

Are you going to play catch-up or feel sorry for yourself? What other things are you doing to make sense of your life now?

I spoke to many patients at different stages of their illness and it became clear that there were varying levels of concern in those who had been diagnosed. For some men it seems, prostate cancer is no big deal, for others it is a different story but I am not referring to attitude here; the variance I am concerned with is due to other reasons. It is absolutely true that attitude plays a huge part at all levels, but other factors alter the starting point for all of us.

There are degrees of seriousness with every cancer and it is just the same with PC. Some men are affected less so and some more so. Those affected less are likely to have been diagnosed at a very early stage, or their cancer is a low-grade type and could be a virtually benign or harmless cancer. For these men, there is a higher percentage chance of complete recovery, or at least living out a longer life without being affected by PC.

Older men, say 70 years onwards, developing prostate cancer are mostly blessed with a lower grade cancer. If that is your age group, then your likely outcome is that you will expire with prostate cancer rather than from it.

Other cases may be either diagnosed late in the cancer growth process or, it is a high grade and very aggressive type, which increases the likelihood of it having set up home elsewhere in the body, reducing the chance of a full recovery. A cancer that has spread is much more difficult to treat than one in its initial location only.

These are all still prostate cancers but the predictable outcomes are so far apart that a lot of confusion is caused when the subject is discussed with patients. What counts for one case does not count for the next case.

Whatever your position may be in the above scale of seriousness, I will deal with positive help further on.

Speaking with and observing other patients, it became apparent that under the quiet calm exterior most were displaying, was a mixture of bewilderment, fear and good old-fashioned bravado interspersed with splashes of doubt. Anger has been a surprise for me to see in some, I couldn't quite see that. Frustration I could understand, but I couldn't find any anger. What could I be angry at? But that was only my way of thinking, there isn't a right or wrong way to react, nobody is wrong.

Surprisingly others seem to have been brought to life either by the attention they were suddenly receiving or by adopting a very positive attitude and seeing their diagnosis as a new adventure.

This I felt was a good attitude to adopt, unfortunately everyone can't manage that.

Observing the partners of some of these patients told a different story.

The one thing common to most of the men confronted with PC is the lack of knowledge regarding their condition and understandably so. First being plunged into an abyss with the diagnosis, then this life stopping event affecting the family and the compounded effects of all this on work commitments. Finally the realisation that whatever you might be told, it is you who is in there living with and owning this alien process, and even you don't know what the future holds for you.

But then, did you ever? The chances are the clock controlling this PC has been ticking away for years, the only difference between now and before you were diagnosed is that before, you hadn't been diagnosed.

In the normal course of life, those people who don't feel the need to plan their future too far ahead at the best of times, suddenly change their thinking patterns when a threat like this is exposed. Immediately, this life becomes finite; the unexpected awareness that it does actually come to a conclusion, hits home.

The lack of knowledge and understanding at this stage of events can cause confusion for many. It has been voiced on numerous occasions that when major decisions taken at these times are looked back on later, they appear to have been taken too hastily.

Some men, unable or unwilling to be bothered to think about so much at one time, carry on regardless thinking 'it will be alright'. Very often it is.

Unsurprisingly, not being familiar with the medical terminology puts many on a back foot and they become either afraid or reluctant to ask many questions of the various people who are dealing with them. Many of course don't know what to ask and rely on the consultant to tell them all they need to know. This it seems is a common problem. I did just the same at the beginning. At the first appointment, the questions I wanted to ask only came to mind after the appointment was over and I was walking down the corridor on my way home.

That didn't happen again, I did my homework and absorbed as much knowledge as I could under the circumstances, and time available before my next appointment

A word here about the foreign language used to describe medical conditions, body parts and plant-life. It is mostly a mixture of Greek and Latin and used by those in the business the world over. Although many outside of the plant-life or medical business might think it all cumbersome, it makes for universal understanding, a common learning approach and fewer mistakes.

For those of us not medically or garden-ally inclined, it remains one of life's areas of mystery, and some perceive it as an area of secrecy "why don't they say it in English" Think of it as a sort of Esperanto of the medical profession.

I remember being about seven years old and my Dad, who thought this was amusing at the time, was explaining to my mother at home that a colleague of his had a backache, was in some pain and was concerned. He had gone off to his GP who after examining him told him not to worry; he had Lumbago. This formal term issued by a doctor of medicine gave his problem an identity which reassured him and he was then content with knowing that his problem was lumbago, little knowing that the term is from the Latin 'lumbus' meaning loin or lower back. The term Lumbago is really Latin for backache.

This example of giving unwarranted substance to unfamiliar terminology may be from fifty years ago, but in this respect little seems to have changed for a large number of men over fifty, today. Collectively, we as a nation like to give health conditions and even people who have certain health conditions, labels, and then make judgements about them.

Occasionally the one percent of a person who is affected with a condition or difference becomes a recognition handle for the whole person.

Analytical in my approach to any new situation, (I enjoy learning, every day of my life) but not in this case, the first appointment was such a shock event. It was the second appointment onward that I made the most of the opportunity to gather as much knowledge as possible from those with experience.

When I did start to ask questions, I found a willingness on the part of the professionals to answer whatever I asked and if I didn't understand what they meant, I asked again or made notes to research later. I bring this subject up because of all the people I have been involved with on this journey, I found only one person who sounded to me like he would prefer I didn't ask so many questions and that was, I think, because he had what felt like a machine gun up my bottom at the time and was trying to concentrate on taking a biopsy.

I believe that for the most part, with regard to patients and information about their own health condition, the problems they face are mainly within themselves. Their response-ability for their own welfare rates at about four out of ten. Rather than take time and effort to try and understand their own predicament and participate in it, on a regular basis patients readily surrender their bodies to medical staff almost as if they have become detached from their physical selves.

I am sure that if they could, many would say 'ok, I'll leave that with you and call back for it later'

Possibly many people just can't grasp the situation or the complexity of the processes, or they would rather not know. when speaking with them at their homes, they have asked me questions that they should have been asking their consultants. They do want to know more, generally speaking, but won't ask those that have the answers about their specific state and condition, although I am told that this reluctance is declining.

I have on occasions been asked 'why is it, that so-and-so was offered this treatment but I wasn't offered it, why would that be?' The questions may have been asked but the answers not understood. I answered this by saying that some treatments are available to some and not others. Different types and stages of the condition and various symptoms present numerous challenges and require an assortment of interventions.

Working at obtaining explanations for what happens and why it happens, and what options there are, are all part of what we as patients, have to be responsible for.

The onus has to be on us the patient to ask, as there are many who say they would prefer not to know. There is also the stress factor of information overload for many; some people just cannot cope with what seems like everything coming at them at once, the whole thing becomes an onslaught.

How do you rate your response-ability with regard to your own health and that of your family?

Unfortunately for others, due to the state of mind of the patient, when some of the information is passed on, details are missed or forgotten.

By many patients, all that is focused on is light at the end of the tunnel, even though at that point there is no visible light. Little attention is paid to the present moment, and much may be overlooked.

It was announced recently that seventy thousand patients failed to turn up for appointments at the Queens Medical Centre, Nottingham, in the year 05/06. That takes some believing, however I do wonder how much of that is down to patient confusion, fear, apathy or anxiety. It would certainly be enlightening but probably not possible to establish a breakdown of those statistics and find the reasons why.

For those of us who want answers to our predicament but are not sure what questions to ask, I have suggested some of them later on in their own chapter. It is worth remembering that if you do your homework and ask questions that show you are concerned about what is happening to you, you will convey a sense of 'wanting to know' which will elicit more informative answers. On one level, Medical Consultants are no different from anyone else and will respond more positively to you if you sound as if you want to know what he is talking about. This lightens the energy in the room and you will connect better with the person you are speaking to.

Does this sound a bit strange to you? Give it a try the next time you talk with anyone. With a positive attitude, show real interest in whatever you are discussing, and notice the look of engagement on the other persons face.

For the rest of us who know the questions but feel reluctant to ask them, it is time for a change in attitude. Just ask yourself 'what's the worst that can happen, what am I afraid of?'

If you think you will look or feel silly asking questions, ask yourself 'Would I judge someone that way when they were asking me questions about something I had knowledge of and they didn't'. When you have decided that you wouldn't judge someone that way, ask yourself, what makes you think that you would be judged differently.

If this is still a problem for you, pretend to yourself that you are asking on behalf of someone else. This attitude will also be useful to the plentiful supply of us males who really don't like to show our feelings lest we appear weak, or (we think) look silly asking questions, the answers to which will probably confound us.

If the answer to a question creates another question in your mind, ask that one next.

It really is pointless having a consultation and coming out thinking 'I wish I knew what he was talking about' or asking your partner 'what did he mean by that?'

The reality is, these professionals you are dealing with are just other people but these particular other people know what they are talking about on a physical level when it comes to your particular problem. They actually enjoy sharing their knowledge with you if you show an interest, but most are reluctant to impose it on you if you don't.

Don't be on automatic pilot, be sincere and develop an attitude of gratitude to those who are doing their best for you. A positive attitude towards those who are there to help you will make you feel better within yourself for showing this appreciation. Try it and you will feel better for it.

Getting the information from the horse's mouth regarding your condition is essential. It is the only place that will have the detail applying to you.

Other gathered information fills out the bigger picture and gives you a better understanding of what has come your way and where you are on the risk ladder.

Half-truths and rumours are an enemy of those who are ill as they will misdirect and serve only to confuse and undermine those seeking an understanding of their illness.

Good intention and logic tells me to keep all of the subject matter on the upside and deal with matters in a positive frame only, although my heart tells me that as there is so much of the other stuff about, the important issue of misinformation which masquerades persistently as truth should be dealt with also.

Fearing for your future as well as being in a state of anxiety about the present may seem bad enough, but is more so when coupled with a strange environment and the reason for it all is your own illness. Misleading information can increase the negative effects you are already feeling, mostly when the word cancer is in there somewhere.

We shall look at a few half-truths or confusing pieces of information later.

SELF-HELP GROUPS

'questions without answers are within'
ROGER KENLEY DAWSON

SELF-HELP groups are springing up in many places for PC patients and for many these are proving to be very beneficial. Sharing experiences whether good or bad lets us see firstly, that we are not the only one with these circumstances, secondly, which symptoms others are experiencing and how they are dealing with them and thirdly, we get to meet others who are further down the path that we may be treading, so potentially we are looking into our own future.

There is nothing to lose in making enquiries at your hospital to see if any groups are formed as yet. If there aren't any, start one, there are bound to be plenty of potential attendees.

Your consultant will be aware of the enormous benefit such a group will bring to the patients and he will be pleased to participate. If there is an odd one somewhere who doesn't want to take part, you may decide to show him this book and point to the previous sentence where it says he will be pleased to participate. If there is still no interest, ask to be transferred to the Nottingham City Hospital Urology Department where everyone is so helpful. Also make sure that invitations are sent out to new patients who have not yet started their treatment. For many of these, having a connection to others who have already been through what they themselves are facing will give them a sense of their new reality.

When I was diagnosed, I was told of a self-help group that met every month or so at the hospital. I decided in my wisdom, that as I have always paddled my own canoe so to speak, I would see things through for myself with the help of those close to me of course. With hindsight, this was probably a mistake but we all have to learn.

Attending such a group would have given me possible insight into my future condition from those already living it, so from a 'patients perspective.'

Having good information available aids treatment and recovery. It is valuable as it puts parameters around the situation and helps to keep things in perspective.

A surgeon or skilled professional who understands the subject as thoroughly as can be expected, is the best place to get the mechanical facts, there is no doubt. He can also give you outcomes and prognosis based on previous experience and data.

Hearing from others what it is like to be on the receiving end of treatment, when you yourself are living with the problem in your own body, helps on a different level.

First hand information from both perspectives puts you in the best position of understanding that you can be in.

I am sure we have all had times when contemplating a holiday in an unfamiliar destination, we decided to ask someone who had visited, what it was like, or heard someone describing where they had been and thought the place was worth a visit. From that, it is easy to see that we can all take comfort from the experience of others. When you give it some thought, we habitually draw knowledge from the experience of others, so why not do the same thing where our health is concerned.

Maybe it isn't quite the same thing as asking a gardener about how we can expect a certain plant to grow, or a mechanic about any problems we might anticipate with a particular type of car, but if we choose to treat it in a similar way, we can quickly learn and come to terms with it and by doing so chase away the fears.

Listening to, and learning from positive views of another can quell many of the unwelcome feelings that accompany the journey we are on.

LIFESTYLE

'Look at yourself in the mirror, do you see a grape, an egg or a coconut.
Now look for yourself, find the grape.'
ROGER KENLEY DAWSON. FROM 'THE SHELL WE FORM'

THERE are many books available on the subject of PC and many make interesting reading, full of detail and theories as to what triggers cancers.

Theories with regard to causes are often analysed in detail, frequently claiming to explain why men who include this or that in their diet or have a certain aspect to their lifestyle are more inclined to get PC.

Because of this approach many men, encouraged by their family who want them to be around for longer, are press-ganged into altering their lifestyle and diet, sometimes quite dramatically.

Making severe changes to your lifestyle in ways suggested by some campaigners may cause such a shock to the system that any anxieties or symptoms of your illness pale in comparison.

I vividly recall the initial days after diagnosis and my reaction. Accepting this new reality and attempting to soak in all the information available and make sense of it all was overwhelming. Don't eat this, don't eat that, alcohol is the cause! Dairy produce is the cause! All at once it appears that everything you have been doing for the last thirty years has been bad for you and you are the architect of your present condition. I don't really know now whether or not I have been the architect of my condition but what I do know is that whatever the cause, it hasn't happened overnight and it isn't going to be undone in a month.

Careful thought needs to be given before any changes, I'll go into this in more detail, later.

I did ask at one appointment that 'as it could be determined how much longer it would be before I would have a serious problem were I to choose to have no treatment, could it also be worked backwards to see when it had all started'. The answer was 'no it couldn't. It doesn't work like that. It may have started even before you were born'. With that answer and at that time, I started to wonder whether the cause to this challenging condition was generated in this lifetime, or was it in a predetermined life plan over which I had no control. Continuing in my eagerness to find a solution and beat this cell corrupter, I continued to scour the Internet and talk to as many men with this condition as possible.

I believe that when told that it may have started before I was born, the meaning was behind it was, there could have been a precondition, increasing the risk of me developing PC.

Looking for help through the various websites at that time, I saw that there was much mention of a substance called 'Lycopene'.

Lycopene, wait for it, is an 'open-chain unsaturated carotenoid. It is a proven anti-oxidant that neutralises free radicals' In other words Lycopene is claimed to zap malicious entities that are thought to cause cancer and are circulating in our body. For many years now, Lycopene has been recommended by renowned scientists as a vital ingredient to consume in order to avoid various diseases.

An experiment carried out in America at the University of Toronto, entailed doses of Lycopene being prescribed to half of a group of men who had all been diagnosed with prostate cancer by biopsy. The Lycopene was given to the men after they had their biopsy but over a period of six weeks before they had their prostatectomy. The other half of the group who had also been diagnosed by biopsy was given nothing during the time between biopsy and prostatectomy. After the whole group had their operations, the tissues removed during the operations were compared with the tissues removed during the biopsies. It was claimed to be that the cancer cells in tissue removed during the operations from the men who had been taking Lycopene had a reduced further deterioration in the cell structures than in those taken from men who had not taken Lycopene. The conclusion drawn from this was that the effect of Lycopene slowed the progress of prostate cancer in those cases. Consuming Lycopene therefore, may slow tumour growth or be a likely preventative measure against developing the condition.

At that time, I was looking for instant results with anything and everything that had been remotely associated with curing prostate cancer, so much so, I was eager to start swallowing anything that was claimed would be beneficial to me, irrespective who was doing the claiming.

Lycopene is present in various vegetables such as red peppers and carrots, watermelon and pink grapefruit. As I write this, I hear pomegranates have also been added to the list. It is the red colouring or the chemical that goes to make the red colouring.

The write-up claimed that the best place to obtain Lycopene is in tomatoes. Reading further I found that raw tomatoes are not an option as our digestive system cannot extract the substance from raw tomatoes, instead they have to be cooked at high temperatures to release the chemical. Tinned tomatoes were rated better than cooking them at home, but due to the very high temperature reached in processing, tomato ketchup was deemed by far to be the best source of Lycopene.

I went to the cash and carry outlet the next day and bought catering size bottles of the stuff and for about four weeks drank a cupful every day. The first day or two was a new experience, as I had not eaten tomato ketchup before; after that the sense of purpose took over and I continued to drink it daily.

After four weeks or so, I came across a website that drew attention to the information relating to Lycopene. It stated on the website that the actual study into Lycopene was in fact funded by 'Heinz' the food manufacturer and commented that the funding source may have influenced the outcome of the experiment.

If the circumstances were different, this could be funny but when it is concerned with serious health problems, it isn't.

Checking the facts, I established that 'Heinz' did fund the experiment. If you take a cynical view, this could put doubt into your mind regarding the outcome of this experiment and more besides. One thing is for sure, that it goes some way to let you see how information could be manipulated and distorted to take advantage of people who are looking for solutions to their health problems. It did serve to make me more analytical when looking at other substances that have been given the status of 'aider or abettor of cures'.

The latest claims for Lycopene are that research suggests it is associated with reduced degenerative disease such as cancer of the lung, bladder, cervix, prostate and others. It is also being looked at with regard to the fight against breast and digestive tract cancers, the latter being a scarce cancer in Italian men who are known to eat high quantities of tomato products. Lycopene has also been proclaimed to be active against osteoporosis, heart disease and other conditions relating to ageing. Continuing to read the positive attributes given to Lycopene, it is starting to sound like a 21st century universal remedy.

The reality is that many studies have involved Lycopene and the information from all of them claim some benefit from it with regard to cancers and particularly prostate cancer.

The way some companies, past and present have and do use false claims for health benefits attributed to their products, even in suggestion, as a marketing tool ought to be criminal activity. In a capitalist or free-market system as ours is, it appears not to be, at least not until the false claimants have made their money out of it.

With regard to cures for PC, it is open to the individual to come to their own conclusion. Our bodies are designed to mend themselves naturally but become overwhelmed with our lifestyles, some aspects of which are not easily avoided. The line of thought in medical circles is that the way forward is the genetic route; that is to say from a medical standpoint, the causes cannot be eradicated so let us block the effect.

There is no major gene that is standing out to claim responsibility so the task facing those who are searching is going to take many years of painstaking research. Even then the signs are that there will be no single path forward; many treatments will be needed to deal with the variations of type of PC. The cause of PC is certainly not genetic but it seems that going in that direction will provide a solution more easily than tackling the true causes. The downside to this is by taking that path will take attention away from determining the causes and eventually those same causes will erupt as some other condition.

I have no doubt that the potential for cancers occur in each of us every day. What our body is designed to do is deal with these cancer start-ups with action from our immune system, when this does its job properly it eliminates any wayward cells. It is when our immune system is overloaded with demand for action in other areas or is subdued due to a state of mind, that cancer gets a hold and grows beyond the regular scope of our immune system.

I have no medical or scientific training but what I do know about is negative states of mind generating negative energy that undermines an immune system. Our state of mind is within easy reach and so is within our power to change. Conditioning our mind to generate positive energy will stimulate our immune system to work as efficiently and effectively as is possible for it to do.

WHAT IS CANCER ANYWAY

MENTION cancer and the very word frightens the life out of some people. It has become the 'BIG C' the 'DREADED LURGY' and 'IT' as in 'HE'S GOT IT', in fact any number of euphemisms.

Thinking about it, why shouldn't it frighten the life out of people, it can strike anyone out of the blue at any time. The truth is, even if we are constantly having sonar scans and other medical investigations, none of us ever know what process is beginning to be out of control inside our body.

In spite of all the very excellent equipment that is constantly being refined and upgraded, there are limitations as to what can be achieved. We should be in awe of what has been created in technology over the past thirty years or so, especially in the medical field. Machines are so smart they can produce a three dimensional version of our internal body systems on a television screen. These are miracles of technology that represent scientific excellence and yet there is so much more to be explored. So many forward steps have been taken but there are many more to take and limitations are with us for some time yet.

Instead of being impatient with the speed of development of technology and the expectation of instant cures, a more positive approach to life might be to pay attention to what we are doing that is making us ill, in order to change what we do and avoid becoming ill. We should live more in the moment and be moved to be appreciative of every carefree day we enjoy, carefree in the sense of being disease free; if not disease free then mobile and sane. Learning to appreciate these things may make us take notice of what we are doing to ourselves and to the environment on a daily basis. Perhaps we move more out of habit than thoughtfulness. We ought to pay attention to the fact that all of our actions have reactions and all of the effects we experience have a cause.

According to which article you read, statistics do vary regarding cancers. One thing is for sure, at least some form of cancer will affect one in three men over the age of fifty and as it stands at the moment, PC will affect one in eleven men.

These numbers are currently correct and known to be rising at quite a rate; a portion of this increase could well be due to the ongoing improvement of methods to detect cancers. A larger part of this increase must also be attributed to other material causes such as the chemicals used in modern farming methods for instance. Chemicals used for pest control are poisonous and are sprayed on the crops we eat; the discarding of prudent farming methods have allowed the essential minerals to be stripped out of the soil. The processing of foodstuffs and manufacturing of household goods all involve the use of unnatural substances, which are chemicals concocted by man.

If we add the effects of the lack of minerals in our foodstuffs and the plethora of unnatural chemicals in our midst together, it is easy to see that our immune systems are fighting on two fronts, being undernourished and overloaded. These items all play a part in changing the makeup of our body, and it is likely that these unnatural chemicals are responsible for many of the poor health conditions we are experiencing in the world today.

When looked at in isolation, cancer statistics are quite alarming, but don't overlook the fact that vast improvements in detection and treatment are to some degree countering the increasing impact of cancers, particularly PCs. Had the advances in cancer screening methods and treatment not been made, the statistics would be considerably worse.

The word cancer is a term that has become synonymous, particularly with elderly people, with death. This is because people do die from cancer sometimes, and the longer you live, the more people you will know who have died from all sorts of things including cancers. Cancer deaths can be very distressing in some cases for the families of those affected. It is easy to see why cancer has its reputation.

Years ago, not so much was known about cancer, the technology hadn't been invented to seek out the changes occurring in our bodies as we develop problems. If someone developed a lump or started with a cough they couldn't get rid of, the chances are they were on their way out.

It is now known that many types of cancers exist. I read only recently that there are at least twenty-eight different types of breast cancer. Each of these may have different triggers that activate them.

Some types of cancer are treated successfully, others managed quite well, and some are not.

So much for the bigger picture, now let us look to cancer itself and if you want an explanation in the simplest of terms, this is it.

Our body cells renew on a regular basis and as there are billions of them, there is a lot of activity going on continuously in that respect. As with everything in life, the more occurrences of events, the more chance there is of something going wrong. Occasionally the renewal process of cells go wrong, is not picked up by our immune system, gets out of control and we end up with an ongoing corrupted process. This is what cancer is.

Standing further back from a situation puts it in a different framework and offers an alternative way to understanding. We can use this opportunity to understand more about ourselves as a whole person rather than just the bit with a cancer. One or two people I have spoken to about their condition have listened to the following life view and changed their outlook about who and what they are. They now have a deeper understanding or objective view of their illness and indeed themselves.

The following story may seem a little strange if you haven't given too much thought before to your life. You may see yourself in a different light or it might give you a new perspective on your sense of being. Whatever you think is correct for you but give this some quiet thought.

First ask yourself this; Am I the same person now that I was, say twenty years ago.

Now answer this honestly before you go further.

The usual answers are yes or, more or less or, I think so or, well, a little wiser maybe.

If you think the answer is a yes, point to any part of you that you say is the same as it was twenty years ago.

Wherever you have pointed to, you will soon know differently.

Looking at what a human being consists of will bring some clarity to what we are talking about and it may bring to you a different sense of awareness of self if you apply each of the qualities to yourself mentally as we go through it, take your time and think as you go.

Whoever or whatever you think you are, you actually consist of the following: Within you, is an assembly of memories, whether recent or distant, they are all memories. There are familiar thought processes that you have learned with strong cross-reference links to each other, along with the bias-controlling mental filters that you have installed as you have gone along your life's path. There is also the characteristic behaviour pattern, which others will recognise as yours. These combined qualities create the personality and character that is you. These are completely intangible, as they have no physical matter.

This assortment of qualities is real to you and to those who know you but are quite distinct from and stored in, your physical body.

Your physical body is a food-processing machine that exists in order for your brain, or personal management system, to be nourished so enabling your physical life to continue.

All right so far?

Your body consists of trillions of cells and is in a constant state of repair, a bit like the Forth Road Bridge. Every single one of your cells is programmed to last for so long and then to die, your skin cells for instance last only about three weeks; each cell is programmed to replace itself and is also programmed to die. Every single cell contains a switching mechanism that causes this to happen. This constant process is happening throughout your body all of the time and that is why in reality; you are not the person you were ten years ago. During that time, the majority of your cells have renewed many times over, others have replaced themselves less often, but you have in a physical sense, been completely renewed many times. If all of the cells that have been produced by your body had been saved in their entirety, in theory there would be many physical versions of you all at different stages of your life.

The one you are currently, is just one of those many.

Another way of looking at this is to liken your body to a football team, let us say 'Notts County'. They have been in existence longer than any other league team. During the lifetime of the team, the components, in this case the players, managers and staff, have changed many times, but the team has always been known as Notts County. The team has always kept its identity but it has renewed its make up many times. This is how our physical entity functions throughout our life. When there are many billions of cells constantly renewing and dying, it is reasonable to assume that an error will happen from time to time, and sure enough, it does.

The term cancer here is used to describe the process in our body whereby a cell, instead of renewing and dying, does not die but the replacement process still occurs. The switching mechanism fails and the old cell doesn't die. Duplication occurs and where there was one cell, there are then two cells, these two become four, four become eight and so on. The cells around the corrupted cell also become affected and begin to react in the same way. The area this is happening in soon becomes very crowded. Where home to a few cells were, there will be millions. This continuing duplication is regeneration out of control. The more aggressive the grade of cancer or corrupted the cells become, the more the corrupted cells will affect the adjacent cells spreading the pattern of degradation.

The corrupted process develops at varying speeds according to the type of cancer it is and other factors within the person affected.

Eventually there are huge numbers of cells occupying a space meant for a few.

If the change hasn't been detected by then it soon will be. If on the surface of the body we feel it or see it as a lump or distortion of the area. If the change is internal, the chances are that a function of our body will be interfered with. Early attention is essential otherwise the opportunity arises for a cell or two to break off and travel through the blood stream or lymph system to other parts of the body, setting up home elsewhere and corrupting other cells. If this happens, the situation is more serious, as secondary cancers (metastasis) are usually in a vital area or main organ of our body.

Cancer starting off in or near a main organ or sensitive area is likely to alert us to the change by discomfort, pain, or a change in a bodily function.

An incessant itch or blood coming from a place it didn't use to, or nodules appearing where they shouldn't be are indicators, but not necessarily a diagnosis of cancer.

More than a million people in the UK are known to be living with some form of cancer. They go to work and enjoy their lives to their own comfort level, some excelling more in life than they did before diagnosis, spurred on by the sudden knowledge that their physical life is finite, it really does come to an end.

Each day we wake up is a bonus most of us take for granted until we have reason to think otherwise.

There are many people who are walking about with a cancer and don't know it yet. In many cases, it could be years before their particular problem becomes troublesome enough to motivate them to seek help.

To sum it up simply, cancer is the corruption and uncontrolled multiplication of cells. It can occur in any part of the body, at any time.

It is not known what the fundamental trigger is for many cancers but what is known for sure is that where there are known contributing factors for certain cancers, exceptions create anomalies.

Smoking cigarettes causes lung cancer, but the 100 years old war veteran interviewed on the evening news some years ago swears that his age and good health are due to his smoking 60 woodbines a day for 85 years. There are still people who would say this but such a report is not now considered appropriate viewing.

Many male non-smokers in their mid-fifties who have developed lung cancer in recent years are plumbers who, during the early years of their trade used asbestos cloth as pipe lagging, winding it around pipes in enclosed areas and breathing in the dust. Asbestos dust is a proven trigger of lung cancer. With many cancers now, the type can be established and used to identify the trigger.

To give ourselves the best chance of avoiding developing a cancer there are certainly things that we shouldn't be doing to our bodies, mostly it is common sense.

Burning our digestive tract by consistently pouring strong alcoholic drinks or hot drinks down our throats may cause us to have mouth, throat or stomach cancers developing later as often happens with smoking, now proven.

It is becoming increasingly accepted that many of us have a predisposition to developing cancers, as we have for other conditions. Our genetic make-up, being the blueprint for our physical being, can show whether or not we have a bias towards developing certain conditions, many being cancers.

As research continues, it is becoming clear that some families have an inbuilt genetic predisposition to developing certain types of cancers. This is nothing to do with hereditary cancers. those types are very rare.

When a parent develops certain cancer types, there will be an increased likelihood that the child of that parent may also develop a similar cancer type. This is due to their being a predisposition or weakness, I prefer receptiveness, in the genetic makeup of that family line, PC is in some cases subject to this type of continuity. Whatever may be said about the genes and the predispositions, for the major part, it is our lifestyle that triggers the start of disease.

It is also evident that in some cases, a person's genetic form may carry a weakness that gives a predisposition for developing a cancer if certain conditions are prevailing, such as an aspect of lifestyle or exposure to causation factors, a prime example being a plumber as mentioned previously. Not all plumbers who handled asbestos cloth will develop lung cancer, but those with a built in predisposition will.

With some forms of cancers, there are changes that occur in bodily fluids and processes. These types do not have tumours as such.

A male has a one in eleven chance of developing prostate cancer but if like me, your father has or had prostate cancer, your chance of developing the condition increases to one in six. If your father and a brother have prostate cancer, your chance increases to one in three. I have five grandsons aged eleven and under at the current time, I am supporting the prostate cancer cause wherever possible. You have done so too by purchasing this book. A surplus from the sale is going to prostate cancer research. Thank you.

There are volumes to write about cancer but for our reasons here, there is no point. If we move to the next chapter we can focus on the prostate, it's location and function.

PROSTATE. WHAT, WHERE, WHY.

'Man's mind stretched to a new idea never goes back to its original dimensions'
OLIVER WENDELL HOLMES

THIS mysterious trouble causer seems to have come to the fore of late as the location for the biggest threat to male health in the Western world.

Let us be sure of what we are talking about, it is definitely prostate, even though I have heard it referred to as prostrate and I might whisper this, by one or two medical people.

The prostate gland is definitely a man thing; a woman has no prostate gland.

On average the prostate is sized from as big as a walnut to as big as a large egg and is situated at the neck of the bladder.

It is of a muscle type consistency, is encased in a capsule and is smooth when in excellent condition.

The tube that you pee out of comes from the bladder and passes through the prostate gland, then down through the penis.

Also passing through the prostate are the two tubes called seminal vesicles, they are used to deliver sperm to the penis from the testicles. When having an orgasm, the sperm, produced in the testicles, travels through these tubes to the prostate. As the sperm passes through the prostate, a liquid called seminal fluid is produced by the prostate and is mixed with the sperm assisting its passage to its intended destination, the female egg.

The prostate plays a fundamental role in our regeneration but for many, causes a lot of trouble along the way.

As a man ages the chances of his prostate gland causing problems increase. Infection and inflammation are common conditions that are persistent and very debilitating.

The symptoms of inflammation (prostatitis) and infections of the prostate are quite depressing; the causes aren't known and the conditions are very difficult to treat. The denseness of the prostate tissue makes it difficult for antibiotics to penetrate the area. Symptoms vary in range and intensity, with burning sensations when passing water, as if sitting on a hot tennis ball or, weakness and tiredness; for some the severity may cause feverishness or leg weakness. Treatment usually consists of long courses of low dose antibiotics along with feet-up rest; if left untreated the symptoms do tend to pass but it isn't usually very long before they return. It is unfortunate but once a weakness has been established, problems tend to be recurring for those who are susceptible.

As men don't appear at the GP.s surgery until the situation is more serious, the numbers of men affected are difficult to gauge but due to this known reluctance of men to seek treatment it is known to be a very widespread problem.

Enlargement of the prostate (benign prostate hypertrophy or BPH) will eventually cause continence problems but is treatable. About a quarter of men over sixty-five have moderate to severe symptoms connected to this condition. Enlargement of the prostate will either compress the pee-tube (Urethra) so interfering with the outflow of urine, or enlarge upwards into the bladder creating a ball-valve effect. This is likely to prevent complete emptying of the bladder and can cause bladder infections.

The treatment for this is to remove part of the prostate usually through the Urethra by using a cutting implement called a resectoscope.

The worst of the problems of course is cancer of the prostate.

PROSTATE CANCER

'The journey of a thousand miles begins with a single step'
LAO TZU

THE words 'prostate cancer' for most of us are just another title on a poster in our GPs waiting rooms, and that's only if it catches our eye. Increasingly now though we are seeing similar information-ads in magazines directed at the male population and lately women's magazines; this probably in the hope that, as most men don't take any notice of these things or at least don't apply it to themselves, their salvation will come by the female awakening them to reality.

If prostate cancer is a term you are familiar with, you probably are yourself affected or have someone close to you who is. As is generally the case with most illness, we have little knowledge of it until it appears close to home.

Cancer of the prostate for those not familiar, is like most other forms of cancer, with one exception. It has overtaken heart disease as the biggest male killer in the western world apart from lung cancer.

It is not only affecting more males as time goes on, as mentioned briefly before, but is affecting males of a younger age.

Due to the nature of PC, the earlier in its process it is picked up, the better the opportunity for cure.

The younger the male is when it is discovered, the more important it is to get on top of it. I was diagnosed when I was fifty-five years old and I was told I was young to have this. Young, with regard to PC is considered to be anything less than sixty years.

As well as those who are known to have the condition, there are any number of men experiencing symptoms ranging from stinging when peeing, burning when peeing, having to wait for a flow to start, taking longer to pee sometimes and not others, dribbling after finishing, erectile dysfunction, (medicalese partly for having difficulty getting or keeping an erection), urgency to pee, then nothing much happens, to aching bones and light fever symptoms. So many of us put up with these slowly encroaching changes and think little of them, sometimes with undesirable consequences

No-one knows how many men there are at any one time experiencing discomfort or changes in their urine flow rate. Sooner or later these men will appear at the GP's surgery and only then will they be included in the statistics.

If every man having any of the associated symptoms actually accepted the fact and decided to go to his GP. on Monday morning, it is likely the queues would last for a month.

Prostate cancer is extremely serious and could well be life threatening, but a confirmed diagnosis is not a condition that requires blue lights flashing and emergency 'all hands on deck' type attention. It may feel like that to you, particularly if you are aware of the potential seriousness but in most cases the condition has taken years to get to where it is now. The feeling of urgency is due to the fact that you have only just found out about it. It is quite normal to feel panicky, fearful and anxious, I haven't met anyone who reacted other than in that way when first informed of his condition.

What is needed, just when you feel least able to focus, is a calm mind and cool head. Take enough time to do your homework, learn about the disease, understand what is happening to you, and find out how serious your situation is. Then enquire which treatments are appropriate for your condition and what is available to you. Later on I have outlined some questions to ask when you see your consultant. He will not mind you asking the questions and will be pleased to give you the answers but make sure you or someone with you writes down the answers at the time. Go along to a prostate cancer self-help group for more patient-view information, then based on the knowledge you have acquired, make a decision that you feel comfortable with as to how you want to progress with treatment. Don't forget, it is your body and you are responsible to you for it. Serve it the best way you know how.

Prostate cancer is a common disease in the older male and increasing at a rate not known before. At present, it is recommended that PSA tests for prostate cancer be taken at least every two years once past the age of fifty. If your father or an uncle or brother of yours has prostate cancer, then the age for testing to begin is recommended at forty-five. Personally, knowing what I know now, I would start going at age forty even just to establish a baseline figure with which to compare future readings.

To show how widespread and established PC is becoming in the UK, it is estimated that if all males lived to be one hundred years old, it is probable all would have prostate cancer at that point.

Not so many years ago, prostate cancer was a low-profile condition; treatment was sparse, haphazard or non-existent. As there was no test for the disease and awareness of the now known symptoms was low in the medical profession, secondary conditions developed before any action was taken. Due to the delay in discovering the problem and the inability to treat it, inevitably the patient would die and it was recorded that the patient would have died from what is now known to be a secondary condition. Many deaths are still recorded in this way distorting the true causes of death. If not treated the cancerous process will spread by moving through the blood stream or the lymph system. The liver, bowel, lungs, brain and kidney are common areas for secondary cancers to develop and cancer problems in these areas are more likely to accelerate the conclusion of life.

Biopsy samples can be taken from other areas where cancer has developed and it can be determined whether or not it is a secondary cancer. Lung cancer that has spread from the prostate will still act as prostate cancer and can be identified as such. When the cause of death is lung cancer that started life as prostate cancer, the cause of death should be recorded as prostate cancer. If this would be done in all cases, the true measure of seriousness of prostate cancer in the population today would be known.

My father died from the effects of prostate cancer, he was asleep for much of the last year of his life with leg pain and bouts of breathing difficulty. His cause of death was recorded as pulmonary embolism. I believe this was a symptom of the root cause and not the true cause if the interests of truth are to be served.

Worldwide communication has greatly increased the regular exchange of information from many countries and progressive steps have been made as the wider medical world work on development of prevention and cure for PC.

There is an ongoing prostate cancer study looking into genetic make-ups that show susceptibility for this disease, being conducted by The Institute for Cancer Research & The Royal Marsden NHS Trust. If you are interested in helping our future generations please read the contact information in the Reference section at the back of this book.

There are over one million people in the UK who are living with and managing cancer and accept it as a state of being.

What is this cancer all about? Why is it happening? What is causing it all? There isn't just one answer but as the number of all types of cancers is increasing it goes without saying that it is to do with what we are using, eating, drinking and breathing.

Statistics show that the problem is getting more serious and younger males are developing the condition.

We would all fare better if more information were made more readily available. It is known for sure that causes of disease are pollution, food-stuffs and chemicals in household products. Pollution isn't just air contamination, it relates to toxins sprayed onto farmland and chemicals added to water many of which cannot be removed.

Let's move on to the next section where the prostate cancer symptoms are explained.

SYMPTOMS

*'We do not see things as they are
We see them as we are'*
ANAIS NIN

For our purposes here, a symptom is a characteristic sign or indication, of a state of being which is different to an expected state of being.

If we have a symptom, it is our body telling us all is not as it should be and we need to pay attention to it.

If we don't, the symptom will increase its effect until we do pay attention to it.

Generally speaking, many of us are too busy with things we are concerned with in the present to be distracted by having to pay attention to the minor detail of personal health. Well, that is until a symptom becomes more of a concern to us than whatever it is we would rather be doing. Usually by that time, whatever the problem was when it started, it has begun to affect more of our body than we now prefer.

Symptoms or not sometimes don't mean a lot.

Before describing the symptoms, it is important to stress the following:

While it is true that having any of these symptoms does not necessarily mean that cancer is present, cancer may be present and show no symptoms.

Two or three of these symptoms presenting themselves either intermittently or regularly usually mean there is more of a problem than we would care for.

As men, we should be honest with ourselves but being men even that can be difficult. Tucked away safely in our brain somewhere is an on-board computer management system with an inherent fault that constantly reports back to our subconscious.

The ongoing faulty instruction is that any changes in our bodily functions or noticeable differences in the way we feel will quietly go away if we ignore them.

Any of the following symptoms are an indication that something is not as it should be. They are a warning and medical attention should be sought to determine the cause. Seek medical help if you have any of the following symptoms.

erectile dysfunction

This covers a variety of symptoms but for our purpose here I shall use it to mean an inability to get an erection or to maintain one for long enough to complete sexual intercourse. This is also the symptom that is most noticeable and the one that most men will not want to face up to. The associated feelings of failure and inadequacy affect the male in many ways. Some will even blank the symptom out from their mind.

Below the belt difficulties in the male find their way to the GP. only after an internal struggle. He may find an excuse not to have sex or he may not discuss it with his partner. If his partner tries to make him accept that he has a problem and face up to getting help the chances are he will walk away or pacify her by promising to seek help and then not do so. The difficulty can become so entrenched that sex no longer happens but neither of the couple speak about it. One escape route is he may start going to the pub to save facing the difficulty.

Men who spend evenings in the pub are prime candidates for providing an excuse for not seeking help. Drinking alcohol on a regular basis is known to cause erectile dysfunction and this over many years been called 'brewers droop'. Any malfunction in the erection department of a regular drinker is likely to be dismissed as just that.

If they are lucky, that's what it might be.

The habit of drinking alcohol and accepting the brewers droop excuse could in fact be helping to disguise the onset of prostate cancer. Those who are drinking would point to the alcohol as the excuse for their faltering sexual performance and miss out on the chance to be diagnosed and treated.

Other reasons for erectile dysfunction are furred up arteries, preventing the blood flow into the penis. Diabetes in some causes erection problems. Psychological factors can also play a part in causing this type of problem.

Benign Prostate Hypertrophy (BPH) or enlarged prostate is another cause. It is not cancerous but can cause some distress.

I am sure we all know someone older who takes a long time to pee or has to wait to start peeing, mostly this is down to BPH, but who is to know unless it is checked out?

BPH is an enlargement of the prostate gland. As the male gets older, it increases in size, restricts the flow of urine and can also become so enlarged that it puts pressure on the bladder making the bladder feel full. The flow rate can be reduced to a trickle and in some cases stop altogether. Should this happen, emergency treatment should be sought immediately.

I have dealt with this here, as I want to emphasise the need to determine the cause of the problem as the same symptom could point to prostate cancer.

Erectile dysfunction may also be caused by anxiety or stress but it isn't due to being tired or overworked unless your workload is causing stress.

It is also a mistake to counter a faltering erection with Viagra without knowing why the problem is there. Anyone experiencing erection problems should get checked out for causes before embarking on supplementary action.

Buying Viagra or similar off the internet to enhance failing erections may be serving to conceal the onset of prostate cancer.

Urine flow reduced

This symptom comes on over time and the flow can become quite restricted before we begin to take notice, a bit like looking in the mirror each day and not noticing that we are getting older. It happens slowly and we don't pay attention to it.

If you are not sure whether or how much you may be affected with this, an easy way to measure is; the next time you go for a pee in a public toilet, just take a mental note of how long it takes others to pee. If they are coming and going while you are still there, it might tell you something. If you try and increase the out flow by contracting the bladder muscles and it makes no difference, or very little, get checked out. One patient I spoke to told me he had developed quite pronounced bladder muscles in the form of a hard bulge above the pubic bone and this was due to him pushing harder, probably over years. He hadn't noticed until his consultant pointed it out to him

getting up in the night for a pee?

Well, if you drank a lot the night before that may explain it. On the other hand, has this become a more regular occurrence even when you haven't drunk much the night before? It is usually sufficient to get up once in a night to empty your bladder. Maybe you are getting up more than once in the night; think about it, are you?

finished peeing, do you dribble ?

Can you not quite shut the valve off properly? No matter how much you shake after a pee, you get a little wet patch on your trousers. It never used to be like that, when did that start? Can't remember? Was it a couple of months ago or was it a couple of years? Time flies and you don't take much notice anyway, it could be longer.

No, it isn't anything to do with you being in a rush, is it?

sting or burn when you are peeing, or after ?

Yes it may have happened years ago and it was a water infection, but has it been happening for a while this time and you are sort of getting used to it? Has it become normal, sometimes it isn't there then sometimes it is? Don't be complacent just because it is your body you are inside of and you aren't going to get cancer, because it is your body, and you may do. Be alarmed, seek help.

stinging or burning sensation after sex ?

Is there any sensation of stinging or burning during or after intercourse, now and again or every time? It could be when you try a different position, if that is the case don't decide not to try that position again, instead get yourself examined. Don't ignore it, don't kid yourself any longer that it's just this time it has happened, remember, you said that to yourself last time.

dying for a pee ?

Rushing around looking for the 'gents' thinking if you don't find one soon you will wet yourself. You find one and breathe a sigh of relief, but as you stand there and hardly any pee flows, you wonder what all the fuss was about. "I was dying for a pee and suddenly the feeling has gone"

Wakey! Wakey!

what again ?

'What's the matter' someone says when you are going for a pee, 'you went not long ago, are you alright', 'eh, of course I am' you say, and you think to yourself 'that's right, I did' you dismiss it, but does something niggle? Well it should.

blood in urine

Any sign of blood in the urine and you need to get checked out, even if it's a faint pink colour. It could be anything from a kidney infection to some form of cancer. Don't leave it thinking it will go away.

The following symptoms may not seem connected but they need to be checked out in connection with prostate cancer.

pelvic pain

Any aching feeling in the thighbones, hips, pelvis or lower back.

It could be twinges, soreness or a dull aching discomfort. What about a stabbing pain down the leg, yes, even just once? It could feel like a strain or a stiffness that doesn't seem to go away.

fever/fatigue

Do you start to feel tired when perhaps you didn't used to? After a days work you used to go out or spend an hour in the garden and now you don't because you are tired. Mild flu like symptoms appear from time to time, they don't come to anything so they are not serious enough to concern you. There is just awareness that you feel a bit shivery now and again.

sore prostate with constipation

If you experience a sore area around the prostate, which may feel like you are sitting on a table tennis ball, when you are constipated, get checked out. Countries with the highest rates of prostate cancer consume the highest amount of dairy products but they also have the highest rates of piles. The relationship could be that being in a state of constipation most of the time might be causing aggravation to the prostate. A full bowel leaves less room and puts pressure on the prostate. If this is the cause of continuing prostatitis, a possible outcome might mean a progression to prostate cancer.

other ailment that hangs on

Any ailment that hangs on after you think it should have gone. Yes you might be getting older and you don't repair so well, but as in my case: I developed a chest infection, something I don't normally experience. After appearing at the GP's for a third time in eight weeks, having had two previous bouts and courses of antibiotics, he decided a blood test was in order. That was the start of my journey into the next phase of my life. Any symptoms that appear and don't go in the time you think they should could be a sign, get a PSA test

All of these symptoms are real. They are potentially indicating a threat to your life if you ignore them. It could be so important for you that tomorrow could be your last chance to take effective action. This cancer as with any other cancer moves forward. The more it progresses, the worse your chances of having effective treatment.

Every case of cancer has a start date and a finish date. We don't know what the start date was but we do know that it was some time in the past. We don't know what the finish date is but it is certainly some time in the future. Let us join these two dates with a line. Somewhere along that line from start to finish is a point at which the cancer has had one day too long for successful action to be taken against it, but you never know where that day is. The absolute best you can do is to go along to your GP tomorrow and have yourself checked out.

The above symptoms are a major hurdle for the average male to discuss, especially when they are his own symptoms.

If you are affected in any of the above ways and putting off going to your GP, ask yourself how it is that if your son or brother was telling you these things, you would insist that they were being careless with their lives by not getting things investigated. Now ask yourself, how are you so different to them that this doesn't relate to you. Is it pride or embarrassment or a feeling of failure that puts you off going? Is it that you aren't quite sure what to say when you get there, well eventually you will finish up going anyway, you may as well go sooner rather than later, or too late.

Pandering to your vanity or emotions could be costing you your life.

Be aware that these symptoms also indicate other minor ailments. If there is another reason for the symptom, it can usually be found quite quickly. If it cannot be identified relatively quickly, don't give up on it. Persist with all tests available until the matter is resolved.

Failure to do this may take you on a journey you really would choose to avoid at all cost, if you knew what it entailed, honestly.

If you are aware of members of your family or friends who have mentioned any aspects of the above symptoms, coax them into going to their GP. Sometimes an odd comment or remark may draw your attention, take notice and follow it up with him; without causing alarm get him to take action.

GP'S AND PROSTATE CANCER

'A man is but a product of his thoughts; what he thinks, that he becomes.'
MOHANDAS K. GANDHI

A PARTICULAR type of personality is required to be an effective GP. Whatever else may be in the personality and character of a GP. likeable or otherwise, there needs to be an element of empathy and caring, or it is unlikely they would be in that job. We all know that for the most part do what they can and are of a particular nature.

A GP is a general practitioner. He cannot know everything otherwise he would be a specialist. I don't expect him to be all knowing but it begs belief that there are GP.s in the UK today, who are still not aware or vigilant enough to identify certain symptoms with prostate cancer.

A fellow patient John who was in hospital at the same time as me had been going to his GP over a five year period with symptoms that should have alerted his GP to possible prostate cancer.

John was completely ignorant about prostate cancer, just as we all are before we come into contact with it. He trusted his GP's judgement, as most do. This, granted, with 20/20 vision of hindsight proved to be a big mistake. The prostate cancer had progressed and broken through the gland wall. When past that point, there is no option for an operation and the likelihood is that the lymph system is affected or the cancer has gone into the bones, which is what had happened in John's case.

After my diagnosis, I became concerned for the men in my family and my friends. I harassed them all to go for a PSA blood test. A good friend went to his GP who being well meaning gave him the Digital Rectal Examination (DRE), which entails pushing a gloved finger into the rectum and feeling the prostate through the bowel wall. If cancer is present at an advanced stage, it may be apparent as the gland could have taken on a distorted shape and become hard and knobbly to the touch. His GP said there was no sign of cancer there and everything was normal.

This test is not intended to be a conclusive test for cancer in the prostate. If it is evident that a growth is there, it would already be at the second stage and possibly at a later stage of development. In early stage there are no changes that can be detected by touch. A Prostate Specific Antigen (PSA) test is the nearest reliable test available as a first stop. Had I been visiting this GP instead of the one I was blessed with, my story today would possibly be a different one.

If your GP makes a judgement without referring you for a PSA test, don't accept it, insist on a PSA test. When the results are returned ask what the readings are and compare them with the information in the reference section in this book.

There are some GP.s who think that the PSA test is not a reliable indicator of prostate cancer. Results can sometimes be misleading but it is the best test there is at this time.

It is important to remind ourselves from time to time that GP's and other people we look to for professional support are only other people. Yes they have studied and are qualified and all the rest of it but at the end of the day they have the same life pressures as the rest of us and spend most of their professional lives listening to bad news.

Working all hours doesn't allow them to keep up with what is happening in the outside world and maybe things slip by from time to time. I am not making excuses but we have to be realistic and do the best for ourselves.

The desire to be responsible for ourselves is an individual choice but we need more than ever to be aware regarding health issues. This is not only for us but also for the rest of our family. There is plenty of information about these days; we would do ourselves a favour by learning what is good for us and what is not.

It is our body, logically we should be more responsible to and for ourselves rather than be reliant on others. There are of course things we can't do but I am referring to those things we can do.

Be aware of what your GP.s surgery offers as monitoring clinics and education regarding prevention, take the time to attend and get to know about yourself.

P.S.A.

'Make a living but make a life'
ROGER KENLEY DAWSON

P ROSTATE Specific Antigen is an enzyme that is produced and emitted
naturally only by the prostate gland. It circulates in the blood stream
and is used as one measure to assess the health of the prostate gland.

It was first recognised as an indicator by Dr William Catalona, Head of
Urology at Washington University School of Medicine in St Louis. U.S.
He certainly needs recognition here as his discovery has extended lives for
millions of men.

Prior to this test being used 75% of men diagnosed with PC were at an
advanced stage when first diagnosed. Since this test has been used only
25% are at advanced stage when first diagnosed. Although discovered in
1986 it wasn't used in Europe on a wide scale until 1989.

PSA testing is far from being a perfect test but is the best indicator available. Usual or normal levels of PSA in the blood are reasonably consistent
in males with healthy prostates. From about forty years of age, levels of
PSA in the blood start to increase and continue rising with age. Graphs
are available that show the expected usual levels at all ages. These are true
for the majority of men but there are exceptions.

Raised levels of PSA compared to known usual levels indicate a possible
problem with the prostate and further investigation is always advisable. It

is usual to take two or three blood tests over a month or so as PSA levels increase for other reasons which are not problematic and it is important to discount these. Some other reasons for increased levels are, moderate exercise, cycling, ejaculation or taking certain drugs. Other related reasons for increase are a kidney or bladder infection, recent digital rectal examination, non-cancerous enlargement of the prostate or recent treatment to the prostate. Some of these affect the PSA level for forty-eight hours or more so it is important to exclude these temporary increases.

There are irregularities with this type of test. In some cases prostate cancer may be present with PSA readings showing normal, other cases may show a sky-high reading with no cancer present.

Because of these irregularities, when what are known as false positive readings occur, some distress is caused unnecessarily to men having biopsies, this has to be weighed against men not having the biopsies. False positive readings are readings that show a positive indication or raised PSA level but no cancer is present as proved by biopsy.

At the other end of the scale some cancers are missed due to false negative readings. False negative readings are negative readings showing no increased PSA levels that prove to have been incorrect when later, symptoms occur and a biopsy proves cancer present.

On average just over thirty percent of biopsies taken on the strength of PSA readings show no cancer. Some types of prostate cancer show neither PSA increase nor symptoms.

It can be seen from the above why some GPs do not accept that the PSA test is a credible test for cancer, the point remains there is no better first indicator.

The inconsistencies with the PSA test are on a par with the readings of tests for cervical cancer and I don't think that women, even with knowing this discrepancy, would decide not to have their test.

Prostate tissue is the only place where PSA can originate. After stage one or stage two treatments, either by prostatectomy or radiation, PSA will still be in the bodily system so will present a reading from a blood test for up to three months.

Once test results have shown zero PSA present, a future test showing PSA presence usually means the cancer has returned or more accurately never completely went away. Additional treatment or management is then an option and PSA testing will be used to monitor progress. If the cancer does reappear and it is elsewhere in the body, wherever it may be, it will be identifiable as prostate cancer.

Post treatment PSA testing is often a distressing experience for the individual. After initial treatment the patient is on tenterhooks, his anxiety stemming from wondering whether his treatment has been successful. Usually after stage one or stage two cancer treatment, which is anticipated will eradicate the cancer completely, PSA testing begins with three monthly intervals. For many, the anxiety of follow-up tests begins a couple of weeks before the test day, that day to some degree, resurrects within the patient the original trauma of diagnosis. He is also aware that the presence of PSA can only be measured down to one tenth of one per cent so it can never be said for certain that the cancer has gone completely.

After the blood is taken, there is a further anxious wait of up to fourteen days before he is told of the result. From the point of view of the Consultant, each test that is clear is a good indication that all is going well, and he is probably correct. From the patient's outlook, each time a PSA test date is approaching, he wonders 'is it this time that there will be a reading.'

No longer on the horizon but available today is a PSA measuring device called PSAwatch. It is a portable machine, which acts in a similar way to a cholesterol-testing machine. Blood taken from a finger prick is put onto a strip, which is then inserted into the machine and ten minutes later an accurate PSA reading is given. This is a tremendous anxiety-reducing piece of equipment that is affordable for any health centre or GPs surgery, as well as the cost of each test being less than half of the current cost to the NHS. Elemental Health Care is selling the machine and the contact details are at the back of this book.

Take this book with you to the hospital you attend and show this section or give the information to someone who will pass it for evaluation to those responsible for increasing patient benefit as well as reducing costs.

This is an invaluable machine for use by anyone on a watch and wait programme. By eliminating the waiting time for a result, the apprehension felt at the time of each test is minimised.

GOING FOR TESTS?

'true peace begins with having an attitude of gratitude for life'
ROGER KENLEY DAWSON

I F you are going for medical examinations or tests and you don't know what to expect or what to ask, it can be quite a daunting experience. Here is a simplified breakdown of what to expect and what it all means when prostate problems are the reason for going.

First port of call will be the GP.s surgery.

When you have explained why you are there, the following may happen but not necessarily in this order. It may depend on your age as to what you are asked but mostly it will depend on your GP. and his awareness.

First your GP. will ask follow up questions, how long have you had the symptoms and what is your general state of well-being; are there other health problems in your family history.

There is no need to be anxious; he is building a picture of your overall situation including any background information, sometimes the answers to these questions can be valuable in pointing to a possible diagnosis.

He may decide to send you for a blood test to measure the level of PSA in your blood. This is an enzyme that is given off naturally by the prostate gland all the time. There is a usual accepted level of this in the blood when things are running normally. If there is an amount above the usual accepted level then it could point to a problem of some sort, but not necessarily. This may sound vague but the test is only a pointer and by itself inconclusive for anything. The usual level rises slightly with age, beginning to rise after forty years and continuing to rise as you get older.

Look in the Reference for a list of average levels at any age. Another test performed by the GP. is a DRE. This is Digital Rectal Examination. The GP. will insert a gloved finger into your rectum to feel the prostate gland through the bowel wall. The sizes of prostate glands vary, but the texture is expected, providing the prostate is healthy. Any unusual feature will be apparent. This again is only a pointer and if all feels good, it still doesn't mean that all is as it should be.

If you have symptoms and had a PSA test showing an increased level, the next test you should have is a biopsy.

This will not be done by your GP so you will have a hospital appointment and experience a rather unusual fifteen minutes.

A biopsy, which means literally 'taking a look at life', refers to taking a live sample from the troubled area and examining it under the microscope to see if there is evidence of anything troublesome. The term biopsy refers both to the process of taking the sample and the sample itself.

Taking a sample from the prostate usually means going in the rectum and through the bowel wall with a hollow needle and pulling 'plugs' of prostate out.

This is done quickly and efficiently with a machine. It causes some discomfort for a few days afterward but what's that if your life may be at stake.

The sample of tissue is examined to see if there are any misshapen cells, if there are the results from the biopsy indicate that cancer is present. They are graded and counted using the 'Gleason' scale. This is a measuring scale named after the man who devised it, Dr Gleason.

It seems complicated when you first here the process but read it a couple of times and it begins to make sense.

The number we are looking to produce is created from two numbers and these are arrived at like this;

The more distorted or degraded cancer cells are, the more aggressive the cancer, so cancer cells are graded from one to five with one being near to normal and five being the most degraded or worst. The biopsy sample is put under a microscope and analysed by the numbers of cells in each grade being counted. The grade that has the most cells attributed to it gives us the first number. Let us say that number is four. The grade that has the next highest number of cells in the sample, let us say grade two, gives the second number. These two numbers four and two are added together giving a score of six, which is the Gleason score.

You may have to read that a couple of times before it sinks in but when it makes sense, you will see that it is better to have a score of 'two and four' rather than 'four and two'.

When you ask for the Gleason scale of your biopsy, ask for the two numbers in order to know the exact picture.

If you are going for an operation to remove the prostate, you will have an MRI scan. This is Magnetic Resonance Imaging. To avoid too much information, it is suffice to say that this scanning process detects different densities of tissue and using a computer can create pictures of cross sections of the whole body. These pictures highlight subtle abnormalities to the degree of differentiating between benign (usually harmless) tumours and malignant (harmful) tumours. The term malignant usually means will cause death in the absence of medical intervention. The machines are bulky and you will lie on a short conveyor belt that will pass through the machine while images are being taken of your body. This process takes about forty minutes or so. The machine is noisy like a very loud woodpecker, of a sort.

There are no after effects and to all intents and purposes the process is harmless.

Bone scanning is another process you may be subjected to.

This is not dissimilar to the MRI scan as far as the patient is concerned but quite different in the way it works.

Again there is no need to know all of the ins and outs of the process, save to say that with this machine you will need an injection of some radioactive material and a wait for an hour while this circulates around your body. This solution is drawn to metabolic activity. Any activity such as arthritis or recent fracture will show up with this scan. Cancer activity in bones that has spread from the prostate is usually in the thigh/pelvis area and will be identified by a trained eye.

If you have had a biopsy then you have had the worst of the tests. The rest may cause some anxiety when you see the machines but they are completely painless and leave no after effects.

SEEING THE CONSULTANT

'Having no education, I had to use my brain'
BILL SHANKLY

WHEN going to see the consultant take someone with you. If the news is good nothing is lost, but if the news is not good you may find you are floating with shock or your mind may go blank. I am sure that at these times most consultants have enough about them to understand that such a shock is confusing to the point that you will not be far off automatic pilot for the rest of the consultation.

Having someone sitting at your side will prove to be more than useful, you see what doesn't help is that being male we often tend to show no outward signs of shock or numbed brain. Because of this there is no body language to pick up by those talking to us and the session may just move on.

After the consultant has finished giving you the news of your condition, he will ask if you have any questions. If you do not go prepared it is unlikely you will think of any until you have left the room. Then you will be saying to yourself, why didn't I say this or ask that.

To avoid adding to the possible confused state of mind you may find yourself in make sure you do the following;

Take a pen and notebook with you when you go to see the Consultant.

WRITE DOWN THESE QUESTIONS BEFORE YOU GO.

Ask whoever is going with you to write down the answers to the questions.

1. What is the Gleason score of the samples?
    Write down the two numbers in the order they are given.

2. How many samples were taken, and in how many samples were cancer cells present?

3. Is the cancer all over the prostate or on one side only?

4. With what you know so far, what treatments are available to me?

5. With the most suitable treatment, will it cure the cancer?

6. How fast will the cancer grow if I choose to have no treatment?

7. When would I know that the treatment has worked?

8. What lasting side/after effects am I likely to experience?

9. If the first treatment doesn't work, are their other treatments I could have?

10. To what degree will my activities be restricted

The relevance of these questions may not be apparent to you at this time but as you come to make your assessment about treatment and give regard to your future health then the answers you will be given to these questions will enable you to make an informed decision.

It is your life and you decide what is to happen with it. In order to best decide which direction to take, you need as much information as possible regarding your condition.

Ask the questions; speak out.

Self-consciousness sometimes gets in the way and stops us asking questions about the tests or our condition, or even expressing the way we feel. It is important to remember at these times whose mind and body it is. Your visit to the consultant, the treatment you are to receive and the consequences of your illness are for you to understand and to live through. Don't feel that your questions sound trivial or insignificant, the answers matter to you even if you are not sure at the time what they mean. Later you will.

Don't stop yourself from asking the questions because you are afraid of what the answer might be, it is always better to know than to sit wondering. Knowledge gives you control, it puts you in a position of being able to make the best decision for you.

Sometimes consultants can seem aloof or not quite with you, don't worry; it is probably their way of adapting to the bad news they are forever dealing with.

I was very fortunate to be a patient of Mr. Owen Cole at Nottingham City Hospital.

SOURCING INFORMATION

'Cancelling junk mail may rob an honest man of his job'
ROGER KENLEY DAWSON

A SOURCE of information for more or less anything these days is the Internet, sometimes called the web and for very good reason, if you are not careful you can quite easily get stuck in it.

There is so much conflicting information available that trying to make sense of it all fills you with confusion. If you insist on using the Internet, do so with care when sourcing information about prostate cancer.

Some American sites are financed by private hospitals that have good reason for promoting certain treatments; the treatment they are advising is one they specialize in and are perhaps suggesting it whether it is the best option or not.

Do your homework before committing to any treatment. Find and ask others who have undergone similar treatments recently and see what they have to say. Visit a self help group.

I have provided what I believe to be reliable sources at the back of this book; even so they vary to some degree with their information so just take them on the basis that you have to start somewhere. If you continue to have difficulty finding the information you need, you can reach me through the contact information I have given; I will try to put you in touch with a reliable source.

MISTAKEN BELIEFS?

'Yearn to learn and fill your head, or unlearn and know the truth instead'
ROGER KENLEY DAWSON

W HEN deciding how to write this book, my intention was to provide only information that is positive and helpful. Due to the prevailing and confusing information surrounding cancers I concluded that it is important instead of leaving out grey issues, to include some of them.

For many reasons, as with all other aspects of life, incorrect information can sometimes outreach and outlive correct information. On occasion, the wrong version tends to make logical sense and is difficult to discount on that basis. Of course there are the hardened cynics who say we are being cheated and that the cures are there but we are being denied them. These voices are often given more room than the voices telling it how others say it really is, so on goes the mistrust.

The Internet carries an assortment of information in a way that never could have been before the Internet was there. More information than ever before is available, the sheer volume can be overwhelming with one version contradicting another. Prominent professors and others are quoted on quite bona-fide looking sites on the Internet to support product sales from other countries. When the quotes are checked out, the relevant person denies ever saying such a thing. Unfortunately as yet, the machinery is not in place for the misquoted to have his 'quote' removed.

The information in this book has come from people I have spoken to personally, from very carefully researched world knowledge and studies, and from my own experience, so I know that what I am saying at least happens in the physical world. I have also included carefully researched and selected issues that should be of concern to all of us.

It might be said that this book contradicts another one. Maybe it does in some respects. I am not a Doctor, I have no medical training and I am only interested in conveying to you information that I know is useful and correct. I do not repeat according to who my paymaster is. My intention is to give you what I know. Too much detail can create a fog or blur the edges so that none of it makes much sense but here is enough for you to start to deal with your new or prevailing condition and I stand by it all.

I don't think there are fixed answers to deal with prostate cancer as people have different ideas about what they want, what they perceive their position to be, and more so what they are prepared to do to change things.

Perhaps it is a good idea not to talk to friends and neighbours about illnesses particularly if you have been diagnosed recently. When it is early days after a diagnosis, there can be a tendency to hang onto the words of others whether they are knowledgeable about the subject or not. Numerous people when told of an illness or misfortune don't just listen to what is being said, in their keenness to help they feel they have to pacify with favourable comment. Any information given relating to another persons condition might be absolutely correct but only when related to the person who had the similar condition, which in reality is quite different to your own. Spoken items whether correct or not may plant a seed in your mind and away your imagination goes possibly down the wrong road. It is of no value to you.

biopsies

There is one particular piece of information that seems to fly in the face of logical sense and I have a problem with this one, even though the medics reassure me that there is no cause for concern.

It is with regard to the danger of a biopsy causing the cancer to spread. A biopsy in this case, involves pushing a fine hollow needle via the bowel wall into the prostate gland, then drawing out a plug of tissue to be examined. Inevitably the puncture bleeds. There will be at least eight of these punctures.

It is difficult to believe that this process does not risk spreading the cancer by allowing corrupted cells to flow into the blood stream. When I have asked the question, on each occasion I have been assured that there is no danger from this procedure. The following might convince some but I'm not so sure.

In 2004, I understand a survey was completed and results released showing a comparison between two groups of men. Both groups were due to have treatment for cancer over a given period of time. One group had biopsies. The other group did not. Over the given period there was no difference between the two groups with incidents of secondary cancers. This was conducted in America by a neutral concern, I have no other information on it and so for me at this time, I am not sure what to think.

While we are on the subject of biopsies, a fellow patient, who was afraid that the biopsy he was to have might miss detecting a cancer, said a rather amusing thing, I say amusing because the same thought stream had passed through my mind when I was in the midst of the uncharted prostate waters.

His concern, said to me in all seriousness, was that to make sure a biopsy gave a true reading, seven hundred and forty six samples would have to be taken of his prostate. He had worked it out using some mathematical formula. I asked him whether he had told his consultant about his, he said he had. I asked him what his reaction was; he said ' He just looked at me'. I really felt for him as he was going through a stage of paranoia, thinking that something may be missed. I was sadly amused as I remembered going through the same thought processes myself. It certainly isn't funny but these things serve as a continuous reminder that as different as we all are to each other, we share so much in our inner selves.

sugar feeds cancer

or 'people who have cancer shouldn't eat sugar' as it makes cancer grow more quickly. Apparently, this started out life in a medical journal when reference was made to a sugar based product that was used in an injection given when a patient was due to have a Positron Emission Topography (PET) type of scan. The injected liquid spreads throughout the body and is absorbed by all of the tissues. When there is a higher rate of metabolic activity, more of the liquid goes to that area. It is the activity that draws the liquid, not consumes it. This highlights the activity on the scan and establishes what could be a problem area.

It is possible that a press reporter looking for a story, turned it on it's head and hey presto; a myth is born, or is it?

Alternative views are based on cancer cells having many more sugar receptors compared to healthy cells.

Theories have been put forward over the years about various foodstuffs causing cancer and sugar has had its turn along with most other things we like to eat. Sugar used in moderation (I prefer to think), is quite safe to consume.

similar cancers are treated the same

This is not the case. For a start, it is important to remember that it is always the whole person that is having treatment. People may have similar conditions but are affected differently. These days there are a number of options available. For some situations of course, there may be only one option, probably because it has been found to be the only effective treatment there is for a particular type of cancer or because the stage of the condition leaves limited choice.

No one knows you and your body better than you so if you are sensible in the way you approach your treatment and listen carefully to what is being said, you can evaluate the options and select that which you feel comfortable with.

It could be that at certain stages of a condition, options are limited and if you are so inclined, you may decide to have no treatment. Older patients with slow growing cancers may decide to leave things as they are. Cancers have been known to stop growing and some of the treatments can be quite searching and debilitating, so a 'watch and wait' approach might be taken. It is always your decision.

you can catch cancer.

Even today, it is thought by many that cancer can be caught from someone else. I wouldn't have believed this was true until a time after my operation when I had lost weight and various individuals enquired about my condition; at the mention of cancer I saw the involuntary recoil of one or two people. To their mind at that second I was a leper but their reaction was from their own fear. That is a short distance from thinking that cancer is contagious. Thankfully, everyone didn't react in this way; the vast majority of people were quite the opposite.

Cancer is not a virus or germ, it is a process, one that is malfunctioning maybe, but just a process. You cannot catch a process. If you have been diagnosed with prostate cancer and are sexually active, it is quite safe for both you and your partner to continue to have sex; in fact I would recommend it. Soon it may become more difficult to enjoy.

There are viruses that are known to cause the development of cancer and you can catch the viruses. The two most common cancers caused this way are liver cancer from 'Hepatitis C'. This is passed through Hypodermic needles that are infected and shared within the illegal drug using community.

The other is 'Human Papillovirus' (HPV). This is passed during unprotected sex from someone already infected. It plays a part in the development of cervical cancer. Although these viruses are known to cause the development of cancers, only a small percentage of those with the virus go on to actually develop the disease.

So now you know that you can sit close to someone who has been diagnosed, you can touch him or her and it is even safe to kiss him or her. The fact is, and I can personally vouch for this, after being diagnosed, there is no better time to be touched and kissed by a caring person, whoever that caring person might be.

good people don't get cancer.

Being up and around again after my operation, I bumped into an old neighbour from where I used to live. Aged about 75, he is alone in the world these days after losing his wife some twenty years previously to breast cancer. I had known him since I was very young. As I approached him, he put his face right up to mine, looked me in the eyes and said 'what have you been doing with your life', this was being said in a judgemental way. I was taken aback at first thinking what a strange thing for someone to say to me. It did actually make me stop and think about what I had been doing with my life. As well as working relentlessly for myself in various businesses, I was heavily involved with my community and in a very committed way. I know that my workload could not have been doing me any good really, and I would not give so much of myself in the future. But here was this chap insinuating that my condition had been due to some misdeed in my life and this was Gods revenge, conveniently forgetting that his dear wife had lost her life to cancer, unless he thought that of her too.

I have heard it said that some believe their illnesses came on because they moved away from God and I do recall Glen Hoddle, erstwhile football manager for England making a remark about illness and disability being brought about by events in a previous life.

I can't say whether or not this is true, but we should concern ourselves with the now and the future.

Life itself throws up problems all the time one way or another, but my God is a God of love who helps me to get through problems in this life. He doesn't create them.

If you start thinking that you are responsible for your illness and assuming that your condition is punishment for your sins then the feelings of guilt and associated depression will make you feel more miserable than you may do already. Those feelings spread to those around you and don't make for a good atmosphere, which is a vital ingredient at a troubled time.

Some people just will not accept that flesh and bone is vulnerable to unreasonable changes being foisted onto it.

It is exactly that which we need to be aware of as we continually change our living environments. It is definitely true that physical illness can start in the mind but more from energy imbalances and negative mindsets. Abusing our body wears down the immune system more than anything else. They that see illness as judgement for wrongdoing tend to change their mind when they become ill themselves, believe me.

If you might be tempted to give it any thought, remember that first of all you have to decide what is a good person and what isn't in order to draw a line, then decide which side of the line you belong. Don't bother condemning yourself; true saints are few and far between.

cancer is painful

The worst of cancers may well be painful and there are some cancers that offer no pain at all. Often it can be the treatment that is more debilitating than the illness. This coupled to the stress and anxiety surrounding the situation, add up to quite a trauma for some people with particular conditions, and of course the worst news gets most attention and travels furthest.

A lot too depends on pain threshold; we all vary in pain tolerance levels. Any illness brings changes in sensitivities but recent years have brought a deeper understanding of pain control and much can be done to relieve pain. Relaxation and visualisation techniques have become commonplace in dealing with pain relief and serious illness. Acupuncture and energy healing of various sorts are now coming into their own, being accepted into the Western model of bona fide treatment. These 'alternative treatments' have been in valuable use in the Eastern civilisations in some cases up to thousands of years but rejected by the developed? West.

The strongest painkillers are no longer withheld from people in pain as used to be the case.

private healthcare detects cancers earlier.

Most of the private hospitals in the UK use NHS facilities so it is not the case that they have the ability to detect cancers earlier.

This isn't to say that you won't be treated differently when a cancer is detected, but there can be no doubt that the machinery used to detect cancers for those in NHS hospitals is the same as that used by private health care. The other factor of course is the check ups that may come with private health insurance, but if you are keen to keep on top of your health you can conduct your own regular check ups. The elements you cannot do, you can decide to pay to have them done or go to your GP. He should be glad to help; prevention is much cheaper than cure. There are lower limits for cancer detection, whoever it is for, even the scanners in use now can only detect differences when they have reached say half a centimetre or so in size.

Whether you use private health care or not your care starts with you and your awareness of yourself. It is you who has to take yourself to your GP in the first place. Make sure you get the best care available to you, whomever you use.

talcum powder & cancer.

A couple of years ago I read that at the centre of several cancerous tissue samples taken from young women were grains of talcum powder. It was suggested that the talcum powder had found it's way into the female genitalia and had been a trigger for the cancer condition. I don't know whether it applies to all talcum powder but one ingredient used is aluminium and that has been associated with other progressive illness in the human body. There has also been speculation that some ingredients in antiperspirants and deodorant sprays which are designed to put onto the skin, cause cancer. This has been denied time and again by manufacturers, now it has supposedly been proved that these various products are not absorbed through the skin. Well, if you decide to believe that, it is up to you but the skin is the biggest organ of the body and it reacts to its environment. We do know that anything that is put onto the skin is absorbed through the skin into the body. Nicotine patches rely on this happening in order to be effective and people have died from anaphylactic shock by merely touching something they are allergic to.

The official line is 'At this time there is no proven link between any of these things and cancers'. So say the National Cancer Institute of America.

I would say avoid putting anything on your skin or into your body that you don't need to. It isn't that I don't accept the findings from some official sources but, what am I saying, of course it is. I do keep track of misinformation being banded about from our own official bodies to protect business interests.

You may bring to mind the Chernobyl disaster in Russia in 1986. Clouds of radioactive dust drifted all over Western Europe and settled on high ground. Wales was affected and areas were cordoned off for quite some time. Sheep were grazing at that time on that high ground and have done so ever since. Sale of sheep from those areas was banned for a time but now, it is all forgotten about. On the one hand we are told that radioactive material contaminates for thousands of years and plant material takes up some of whatever it is grown in, I do wonder why the sheep have, since 1986 eaten the grass and the meat from those sheep has been sold for human consumption.

Farmers for years were being poisoned with organophosphates, which are present in sheep dip, but it was kept quiet until it got too big to keep quiet.

There are many examples of money being the motivating factor when it comes to accuracy of what we are being told 'officially'.

We are told that talcum powder does not cause cancer; draw your own conclusion about this one.

big drug companies hold back cures making more money from treatments.

After dealing with the last issue, it might seem that we should stand a little further back to assess the truth behind this one.

While money does drive most if not all decisions taken with regard to business direction, there has to be a balancing factor, that being; does the business benefit more in the short term with decision A than it does in the long term with decision B.

There is also the whistle blower to consider.

It is difficult to believe, leaving moral obligations out of it, that any company would want to put a high profile discovery such as a cure for any sort of cancer in a drawer.

I would say it would more likely be the other way round, where there is a claim of a cure being discovered only for it to be withdrawn later as a false dawn.

The prestige attached to such a valuable find would surely be too much for even the most avaricious company to be tempted to conceal, I hope.

The other point of view of course is that no drug company is going to spend time and money working on a cure or treatment that a patent cannot be secured on. They would sooner continue to look in the wrong direction in the hope of finding something that might work and they can own, rather than look in the right direction for something that works but they cannot own.

Profit is the motivating factor for drug companies and they certainly are good at what they do. The NHS is at their mercy with regard to the cost of pills and potions as is evident with court cases currently taking place to determine whether a patient should be allowed to receive a particular treatment that is available elsewhere in the UK.

A big concern of patients these days is the unwillingness or inability of NHS trusts to pay for drugs to treat cancers. When illness strikes and a course of treatment known to be effective, is available to some but not others due to cost, it is difficult to accept and as a result patients are resorting to court action.

It isn't only health trusts acting inconsistently. At the present time, having prostate cancer and living in Wales are not two things that should be happening at the same time. After living there for sixteen years, I escaped from Wales as soon as I was diagnosed.

It is quite sad to think that the Assembly of Wales was formed supposedly to respond more readily to the needs of the people of Wales and here we are years later with one in three cancers detected in men in Wales being prostate cancer, and treatments that are readily available elsewhere in the UK unavailable in Wales.

Only four out of each ten men affected with prostate cancer in Wales are given any treatment in an acceptable timescale. Numbers of men diagnosed has doubled over the past ten years and deaths from prostate cancer are on the increase. All of this and the Assembly still drag their feet over prostate cancer.

The latest available figures show that in 2004 for each 100,000 of the population, deaths from prostate cancer were 28 in Northern Ireland, 32 in Scotland, 34 in England, and 44 in Wales.

GIVE SOME POSITIVE THOUGHT TO
POSITIVE THINKING

'Santa Claus sets a bad example, only visiting people once a year'
ROGER KENLEY DAWSON

WITH the onset of any health threat, adopting a positive attitude is recognised as beneficial and it will aid recovery. When first diagnosed I had to mentally wrestle with this, you see, I have always considered myself a positive thinker, that being the case how come I get this cancer in the first place.

Well after due consideration of what my definition of positive thinking had been and the sort that was being referred to as an aid to recovery, I began to see the light.

During my involvement with community projects, I had periods of severe frustration at times when so many people who are in positions to make things happen choose not to. I hadn't realised in my enthusiasm that if they solved the problems they would be surplus to requirements so they chose to manage the problems.

My style of progressive positive thinking clashed with their complacent attitudes and I would carry the frustrations within me.

My view on life has always been to look for an opportunity, develop the idea, put a time plan on achieving the outcome, then implement action, ploughing on until the plan came to fruition; all moved forward by positive thinking and driven by desire and intention.

It was not until I was stopped in my tracks with a diagnosis that I became aware that I hadn't applied positive thinking to myself on a personal level. Looking in the mirror after being diagnosed I saw myself, but it wasn't the same person I had been seeing in the mirror each day before. I saw the same image but what had changed was the attitude behind the eyes I was seeing with.

When considering other options for treatment one of the treatments I enquired about was homeopathy. I was advised to see a lady in Manchester who had been dealing with cancer patients for 25 years or so and had good results. When I phoned to make an appointment, I got into a conversation with the lady taking the call.

I explained the position I was in and she said to me with an intuitive resonance in her voice 'have you had any fun lately', I thought for a moment or two and said 'no, I haven't'. This was the point at which I knew I had not been paying attention to my life on a personal basis and had been doing nothing to balance life out, so to speak.

I knew from that moment that the stresses and nervous tensions I had put my body through for the past few years had definitely contributed to my health problem. I am not saying it was the cause but I now know that my immune system was weakened by my own failure to notice I had been holding onto negative energy and this coupled with detrimental environmental factors caused my condition.

I immediately started to change my way of thinking about everything. I dropped all that I was doing and decided I wanted a different life. I launched myself into a completely new frame of mind to deal with that which I was facing.

Positive thinking for me was always not accepting a failing situation in any project I was involved with. Any plan or blueprint of a development or business creation had a cost and a do-by date.

By continually monitoring whatever the situation was and applying the plate spinning technique to matters in hand, the conclusion was inevitably reached. A few nerve endings might have been in tatters but I always got there.

This is a very assertive mode of positive thinking and is diametrically opposed to the positive thinking needed to address health issues.

My previous type of positive thinking comes from an inner need, seeded usually from earlier life and not consciously learned.

The type of positive thinking needed to deal with health issues can be learned but is not taught. It should be taught in schools.

By seeing the reality of true positive thinking in the whole picture of life rather than a section of life, I have found a new way to live. I have encompassed positive thinking in all of life's activities and am further developing this approach to life. Positive thinking is a term that is overused and a practice that is greatly underused.

I will come back to this when I have finished dealing with prostate cancer.

THE EFFECT ON THOSE AROUND YOU

'Greens on a golf course are numbered but in nature are without number'
ROGER KENLEY DAWSON

A VERY difficult thing to measure is the effect of a person's diagnosis on their partner and family. When a man has been diagnosed with cancer, those around him are as much in disbelief as he is himself. Those close to him want to say things and don't know what to say, thinking that whatever they say is futile, or it may not quite convey the meaning they had wanted or even that the situation is beyond words. They just wish he would say more than he does, so that they don't have to.

The focus is on the man who is sitting there, but he is a typical male, pondering his position in life, saying very little.

He doesn't want to talk about it but inside his head he is wrestling with this sudden change in his circumstances. Partly, he can't understand why he doesn't feel differently to the way he felt yesterday before diagnosis and this itself adds to the confusion about his new reality. Periods of despondency occur spontaneously. He will stand up and walk around for no apparent reason, body language revealing his inner mental activity.

If we stand back to see what is really happening, it may help.

Let's call the man Joe. He is a normal everyday chap, likes a laugh and a glass of beer now and then and keeps himself occupied. He might have a moan about something or other, maybe once a day. Regularly he can't find his car keys or his shoes or the last thing he had in his hand. Like I say, a normal sort of chap.

Out of the blue or so it seems, Joe is diagnosed with cancer. As with all men, Joe doesn't seem to understand what is happening. He either carries on as usual for a while or he clams up and goes into a trance. He is trying to deal with this thing but first he has to sort it all out, get it into some sort of order. Only then will it make sense.

Being male, there will likely follow a manic urge to rip it out of his body. This might be well disguised but that is what he is thinking.

If an operation were to be offered that afternoon, he would be first in the queue, breathing a sigh of relief.

Joe's wife is Joe's wife. She has been married to Joe for years and is quite used to his ways of forgetting things, blaming her for moving his newspaper when he can't find it, when really he left it somewhere else. She still has a smile to herself from time to time at his manlike behaviour.

Suddenly Joe has become a different Joe, the shock to his system has stopped him doing things he has always done. He has even stopped eating. Everyone feels for Joe, the focus is on him and how he must be feeling.

Lets look at the effect of all of this on his family. His wife not only has to absorb what is shocking news about her husband, she also has to make allowances for behaviour changes and adjustments to all sorts of things. Meals are not regular items anymore. Joe is awake all night and asleep all day. Most of all, she puts her feelings on one side in order to stay strong for Joe.

All of these changes are extremely stressful and the sad part about it all is that so often, there is no one to ask how she is. So occupied with Joe has everyone become, that his wife gets forgotten.

It is the stress of all of this, that at times can become too much for Joe's wife and she just might snap at him because he is getting on her nerves. The reality is of course that she is tired and so sad.

Women are definitely better equipped to deal with these things than men ever are. That doesn't mean they are harder, they are just better at it and for most of the time, they cope well with hiding their feelings.

Offspring, even as adults react in different ways, they might deal with it by brushing it to one side as if it will be gone tomorrow like a cough or headache. They will say things like 'don't worry, you aren't going anywhere'. Unless they have had a close encounter themselves or within family or friend circles, they don't know quite what to say. One or two patients I have spoken to said their children stayed away; probably as a path of least resistance.

It can be horrendous to see not only dad who is now depressed with his diagnosis, but mum as well who is having to deal with it and keep life together.

It is true that some families suffer more from pain and trauma as on-lookers than the person who has been diagnosed.

If you hear of anyone who has been diagnosed with a serious condition and you pay a visit to wish him or her well, remember to pay as much attention to the carer for that person, it goes a long way.

The carer may look surprised with your questions, it is because no one else asks and they feel new to the situation of being asked, even awkward because the questions should be about the one who is ill. Ask, it will give a feeling of support and help to carry them forward.

STAGES

"Is nature or nurture to blame for your wrongdoings?'
Just put your hand up.'
ROGER KENLEY DAWSON

WHEN consultants discuss prostate cancer, they will usually refer to the Stage of the cancer. If he doesn't, you should ask him about it. There are four stages of progress that prostate cancer is divided into. Treatments vary according to the stage of the condition as well as other factors. Knowing the stage of your condition will help you to understand the reasons for the treatment offered.

STAGE ONE

This is the earliest stage in the cancer process and indicates microscopic cancer particles that have been confirmed to exist but cannot be felt. The DRE mentioned earlier would miss a cancer at this stage if it were the only check used.

Operation is available at this stage.

STAGE TWO

The cancer has developed to a size that can be felt but as yet is confined to the prostate gland. The option of a radical prostatectomy is still available

STAGE THREE

At this stage, the cancer has broken through the prostate capsule and has spread to surrounding tissue but as yet is localized. An operation is no longer an option.

STAGE FOUR

This is advanced cancer that has spread to other parts of the body, usually bones or main organs. This is still treatable and can be managed but is beyond the scope of a cure at this time.

SURPRISING REVELATIONS

'Urec, reuc, creu, ruce, eruc, ucre, cure.
Out of chaos can come order'
ROGER KENLEY DAWSON

S PEAKING with men diagnosed with prostate cancer as well as their families, has given me insight into how people have been affected and how they come to terms with their predicament. Gaining their confidence hasn't been easy, but I have managed to collate some quite interesting information.

It wasn't easy, as we are by our very nature secretive about ourselves, especially so when it comes to speaking about matters relating to the penis and parts. Maybe that's a built in precaution just in case the subject gets around to sizes.

There is one thing I want to bring attention to at this point.

One man I spoke to thought that when he was told that the cancer was progressing, he thought that it was getting better. A progressing cancer is spreading not improving. It is interesting to see how we can easily interpret meanings of words and phrases depending on what we may want to hear.

Surprisingly many families tell the same story with regard to symptoms before the diagnosis. The families had noticed changes in temperament and energy in some cases for months or years before a diagnosis of prostate cancer but rarely were the changes seen as symptoms of a health problem, they were just accepted as part of what happens when a man becomes older like the onset of grumpiness. This doesn't mean that all who are grumpy have prostate cancer but often after diagnosis and treatment, many return to be their previous selves, according their partners and families.

In the early stages of disease before we are diagnosed with any specific illness, changes take place in our natural energy. Subtle bodily tensions may occur or our mental capacity may be slightly affected. We rarely pick up these changes as we have forgotten how to listen to the messages our bodies give us.

Behavioural changes may be noticeable to those around us but as we are not conscious of any changes we carry on in our normal way. Others don't associate the changes with anything so don't speak out. Partners who have become wise after the event of diagnosis then recall moodiness, irritability, tiredness and loss of interest in certain things.

If you have had a recent diagnosis, and are interested enough, you might like to ask any colleagues you have worked with or people you see on a regular basis if they noticed any changes in you of late and if so, what were they. I would be very interested to hear what they have to say.

It is only with hindsight that families have associated these changes with the condition but some men have said that before they were diagnosed with prostate cancer, they noticed various bodily and temperament changes within themselves that were unexplainable at the time and they shrugged them off.

There is so much happening in life today and one effect of this is that busy people become stressed and tend to change slightly from day to day in their temperament and their attitude. Work pressures, home pressures, family pressures and financial pressures all heap burdens of responsibility upon us and the changes these bring to the way men behave day to day are seen as normal or at least usual.

Women certainly cope better than men with these changing forces and so generally their outlook is more tolerant in their expectations of their men folk as well as everything else.

Noticeable changes in a person are generally attributable to a particular cause. It is usually obvious why a man has become disgruntled, his car has been scratched, something hasn't gone his way or there has been an attack on his male ego. It is the changes with no obvious cause that I am referring to; these can be changes that happen over time such as weight loss, appetite loss or as previously mentioned, daily approach to life.

You know when you think about it, paying attention to our own body and mind from the inside should be taught at an early age. Signals are being sent all the time from our body and it only takes a few minutes each day to stop and listen to those signals. Initially you may feel this idea is too bizarre, but give it some thought for a minute or two and just think how much trouble we might have saved ourselves if we had done that.

Unfortunately and sometimes tragically, signs become so obvious and troublesome before anyone begins to question the changes, even the person owning the body, that the lives of whole families are drastically changed, all but for listening to the body signals earlier.

One man I recall actually had a sense of relief at being told he had prostate cancer. He said that he knew something was not right, as he had felt at odds with himself for some time. When told of his condition, he suddenly felt better in himself. He said that knowing what was wrong was better than not knowing as it gave him a reason for the way he had been feeling, even though the news was that he had prostate cancer.

Greg, a keen gardener had been experiencing a pain in his thigh while digging. He thought it was a pulled muscle. After a couple of weeks of discomfort, he went along to his GP. He was asked if he had any other symptoms, he said he hadn't but the GP. being one of the thorough varieties sent him for a blood test. Five days later back came the results. His PSA reading was sky high and a biopsy later revealed advanced prostate cancer.

Another man, John, who had been tired and irritable had been putting these feelings down to working hard and being fifty five years old, he assumed that as he was over fifty he should expect to feel tired, due to wear and tear. He went off to his GP for a tonic to re-energise him. His GP, after asking him how he felt and for how long had he felt this way, sent him for a blood test. Raised PSA levels prompted a biopsy, which confirmed advanced prostate cancer.

The case of Mr John Hough, makes very sad reading but is typical of many men affected with prostate cancer. I didn't know John but I did speak to his lovely wife who, at the time of speaking with me was a sixty-seven years old eighty-one years old. She told me that John was a prominent member of the local community in Nantwich, Cheshire. He was a highly qualified railway engineer and was obviously able to organise his life. By looking at how the man was living his life, it would be reasonable to think he would handle illness in a practical way for all concerned.

By the time John was diagnosed, the cancer had spread and it seems, there was not a lot done for him either by choice or chance.

During the years John had the condition, and even when he took to his bed for his last days in 1999, he never discussed his condition with anyone, not even his wife. It is so sad that John was dealing with what he considered a private matter, probably not wanting to burden his wife with something that was essentially his problem and yet by sharing thoughts and feelings through that trying time, both of them would have benefited from knowing that life's events hadn't put any distance between them.

This is so typical of the average male in the UK. Not feeling able to share his troubles with his life partner and often plunged into the need to singularly re-evaluate his life and his values under the pressure of illness.

My own experience was quite a contrast to that which many go through. After two ineffective courses of antibiotics to treat a chest infection, my GP sent me off for a blood test that came back causing sufficient anxiety for him to be chasing me on the telephone three days later. A biopsy confirmed prostate cancer. Thank goodness for that chest infection and for the attentive Dr Pathak MBE for being alert to the signs of a body attempting to overcome a chest infection but unable to do so because of a weakening or energy draining situation elsewhere, a vigilant man.

So, the long and the short of it all as far as symptoms go, is that if any changes occur in the functions of the penis and associated parts, whether it is peeing or to do with the sexual processes, get them investigated. If you are feeling changed, whether bodily or less wholesome in any other way, go and see your GP. If there are no obvious explanations, ask for a PSA test. If your GP doesn't think that is necessary, persist with your request and don't be afraid to ask why your GP doesn't think it could be prostate cancer. A question like that will focus his mind and often change it.

'William Shakespeare 1564 – 1616.
His dash said a lot, what will your dash say'
ROGER KENLEY DAWSON

TREATMENTS & SIDE EFFECTS

' put yourself first without being selfish'
ROGER KENLEY DAWSON

Whatever you may think about your illness or condition, it is important to remember that whatever path you choose to take, it will affect both you and your partner. Don't underestimate the impact that this condition or the outcome from any treatment may have on your lives. It is a physical and emotional journey and a challenging one for both of you. Do your research together, see your consultant together and make the decisions together. You will both have to live with any after effects whether temporary or permanent so it is vital that you share the decision making process.

Don't make any decisions until you not only fully understand the stage you are at with your condition but the likely outcome from any available treatment including potential complications. It is vital that whoever is treating you is someone who is experienced in treating prostate cancer. Don't be afraid to ask what experience s/he has, after all you are entrusting your body to this person and it's the only body you have. The area of treatment is central to where control of basic bodily functions is situated; any or all of these could be affected.

There are a number of treatments available for prostate cancer and as time goes on, new approaches and refinements to existing treatments are being developed.

It is important for the patient to know that all of the treatments are not available to everyone as some of the treatments will not be suitable.

The individual's circumstance will dictate for most part which treatments are appropriate.

Determining which treatment is suitable is not always straightforward; there are a number of issues to consider. Age is an important factor, it is pointless going for major surgery if your life expectancy is short, why take the risk or have the trauma. General health is an important factor, any chronic condition may well have a bearing on your ability to cope with treatment. The stage of cancer will determine the choice of treatments available, for instance if the cancer has spread out of the prostate then there is no option for an operation.

The availability of treatments will vary according to which hospital you are being treated, you will need to discuss with your consultant which treatments are appropriate for your condition and which of those s/he can offer you. If you feel that an alternative would be more suitable for you but is not being offered ask how you can seek other treatment elsewhere.

As well as wanting to know which treatments are suitable for your condition, you need to consider what you want from your life. For instance, if you are seventy-two years of age and your recently diagnosed prostate cancer is slow growing, the chances are you will die of something else before the prostate cancer will affect you.

If on the other hand you are in your fifties and you have the chance of a radical prostatectomy, you may not want to risk being incontinent which is a possibility, or lose the ability to resume a sex life as enjoyed previously, which is probable.

After asking which treatments are possible, ask what effects each treatment may have on urinary and faecal continence and ability to obtain an erection. The ability to control these fundamentals represents a large contribution to quality of life. These basic abilities are taken for granted in the healthy individual but are sorely missed when lost.

Statistics are available to give guidance on many of these issues. High percentages of success rates are fine for those who make up that portion of the percentage but it still leaves the few who are sad and disillusioned with their outcome.

It can be that the more choices available the more difficult the decision; be decisive and do not put off treatment for any reason other than additional health issues. My biopsy gave a Gleason score of six but after having a prostatectomy the true reading was found to be seven. This represents quite a difference and the danger is always that the true reading is higher than that indicated from a biopsy. Watch and wait programmes account for many advanced cancers.

This is not meant to be a thorough look into the technical detail of all the treatments that are available. It is a brief overview of the most common treatments, how they are administered along with the risks and side/after effects associated with the treatments.

Any treatment you may be considering should be thoroughly investigated and understood by you and your partner before going on with it.

Lets now have a look at what is on offer generally.

no treatment

This as an option may sound naive, verging on the reckless or if you have some knowledge about the subject, not as daft as it sounds. As described previously, if you are getting on in years and enjoying good health otherwise and the cancer is slow growing you may decide to leave well alone and continue to enjoy your life.

It could be many years into the future before being affected by this by which time you would probably have died of something else.

It is making a positive decision to do nothing and not to be confused with not bothering to do anything.

This would also be the decision to take if you are already declining with another serious condition.

watchful waiting

Watchful waiting is for a patient of any age whose cancer is believed to be at the low end of the Gleason scale with a low PSA reading. If a cancer progresses, over time it will become more aggressive with a reading higher on the Gleason scale and higher PSA level. The time scale can vary and there is always a chance that the cancer may stop growing, a slim one maybe but it does happen. There are reported cases where a cancer has disappeared altogether.

A period of watch and wait may be considered favourable until the cancer is confirmed to be accelerating, and then select a way to deal with it.

There are many men who choose this method of monitoring and continue to live their lives as normal.

The risks associated with watchful waiting are to do with the methods of monitoring the cancer. PSA measuring and Gleason scoring can both be inaccurate. This means that the cancer may be more aggressive than deemed to be by the measuring abilities available. The cancer could be more advanced than thought to be at the watchful waiting stage and may have spread out of the gland capsule. If this is the case, when the decision is made to begin treatment, it may be discovered that the opportunity for more effective treatment has been lost.

Slow growing cancers can also change quite quickly to become fast growing and if this was to occur soon after a check-up or during a period of complacency when one check-up is missed, by the time the next check-up is due the cancer could have spread.

There is also a condition called 'walking worried', which may affect you. Being preoccupied with your tests and condition may prove to be a psychological burden that may detrimentally affect your well-being still further.

Watchful waiting is certainly not a choice to take in order to put off having treatment.

radiation therapy

There are several variations of radiation therapy. Collectively, it is the use of high-energy radiation from x-rays, gamma rays, and other sources to kill cancer cells; it has been used for decades for treating cancer. It is helpful in that it shrinks tumours, relieves pain from cancer and destroys cancer cells, which fortunately are more sensitive to the destructive effects of radiation than healthy cells.

Treatment with radiation can be given in several ways, from outside of the body, from inside the body and from a mixture of the two. It can also be used in conjunction with other treatments. If we look at each delivery type briefly, you will have an initial understanding of what it entails.

external beam radiation therapy

The beam of radiation is fired from a machine called a linear accelerator. It is vital that the relative measurements of the target area are accurate as the beam can and will damage any tissue its focus comes into contact with. Computer imaging allows the therapist to determine the best position from which to give the most effective treatment and do the least damage to the healthy tissues.

Treatment is usually given daily for five days a week over a period of six weeks. Each session of treatment lasts less than half an hour but more time is spent preparing for treatment than giving it. Being in the same position at each session is vital and various guards put in place to protect areas of the body not to be treated.

The risks with this treatment are bowel problems ranging from increased need to use the toilet to bleeding from the rectum. Diarrhoea, constipation and mucus discharge as well as burning sensation when urinating or ejaculating are potential risks as well as an increased desire to urinate. These symptoms can last from a few weeks to a year or more. For some patients the problems can be continuous.

Erectile dysfunction is a problem with any radiation treatment.

brachytherapy.

Known also as seed implant therapy it entails planting radioactive seeds about the size of grains of rice, into the prostate. This is done under anaesthetic usually on an outpatient basis. Depending on the size of the prostate, up to a hundred seeds or more are feed-planted using hollow needles inserted through the perineum, the skin section between the scrotum and the anus. The seeds remain in the prostate and deliver stronger doses of radiation compared to the external beam treatment. The doses are stronger but only travel a few millimetres from the seed. The dose continues to flow for a few months during which time the patient is advised to avoid close contact with small children and pregnant women.

Candidates for this treatment are those not wanting surgery. The treatment is less invasive with a short recovery time and as radiation kills cancer cells, it is effective.

The risks are impotence and urinary incontinence although they are said to be less with this treatment than with other treatments. The chances are that impotence will not be too much of a problem to begin with and may be alleviated with Viagra or similar. Unfortunately nerves that control erections may be damaged, as may arteries supplying blood to the area, so impotence problems are likely sooner or later.

cryotherapy

This method of destroying prostate cancer cells has been in use since the early 1990s but is still a relatively rare treatment. By all accounts the success rates have been less than encouraging compared to alternative therapies. The treatment entails inserting special rods, again through the perineum, and releasing liquid nitrogen through the rods into the prostate. This freezes the cells in the prostate and destroys them. The amount of liquid nitrogen used is tiny and only small ball areas of the prostate are destroyed at the end of each rod. The rods are moved about using an ultrasound device to track the movement and the aim is to destroy all of the prostate, killing the cancer cells along with the healthy cells.

This treatment can be used more than once and when other treatments have failed. Risks are mainly with impotence. The nerves associated with erections may be lost as they lie alongside of the prostate and as a small amount of tissue surrounding the prostate is destroyed in this process, the nerves become frozen and die along with the rogue tissue. Side/after effects include scarring of the urethra, burning when urinating and incontinence. Pelvic pain and a swelled scrotum are more possibilities but often these subside after a few months.

If you don't fancy surgery or radiation, this could be an alternative.

radical prostatectomy

This treatment is only suitable for cancers still confined to the prostate gland.

It is as invasive as it can get, usually offered to those whose life expectancy is ten years or more and are in a fit state to stand the operation and make a good recovery.

An incision is made from just below the navel to an inch above the penis, the prostate is exposed and it along with the top section of the seminal vesicles and one valve in the urethra is removed along with tissue from around the prostate and the nerves that control erections. The bladder is pulled down and reattached to the lower portion of the urethra.

Sounds not too bad when you say it quickly but the operation can take up to four hours and to be successful requires extreme skill on behalf of the surgeon. A hospital stay of about six days is usual and full recovery can be expected in from six to twelve weeks.

If you choose this treatment you would be well advised to do pelvic floor exercises for three weeks leading up to your operation day. It strengthens the muscles operating the stop valve contributing much to the regaining of bladder control after surgery.

The risks are plentiful; from the operation itself the dangers are heart attack, stroke, blood clots in the legs, infection at the site of incision and death (about 1%).

After effects of this treatment depend on the skill of the surgeon for the most part, but include impotence (mostly), incontinence from temporary to permanent, and a small risk of damage to the rectum. This can usually be repaired with surgery if necessary.

The aim of this treatment is to completely remove the cancer and will do so if the diagnosis was correct and the surgeon is accomplished. If this fails, other treatment can follow.

hormonal therapy

Some types of prostate cancers are stimulated by the male hormone testosterone and as some cancers actually thrive on this, one available option is to starve the cancer cells of the hormone. This is an effective form of management, at least for some time, when the cancer has extended to the outside of the prostate. A hormone production-blocking agent is given to the patient to suppress the production of testosterone. The testicles produce most of this hormone so if the patient has difficulty taking the medication, one alternative approach would be to surgically remove the testicles, ouch.

With prostate cancer there are usually Hormone-sensitive cells and Hormone-insensitive cells. By suppressing testosterone in advanced cases the Hormone-sensitive cells will die and the cancer will be held in check or reduce. After a while the Hormone insensitive cells will begin to proliferate and grow unchecked.

Hormonal therapy is also used with other treatments. It may be used to shrink the prostate and tumours before giving radiation, making treatment more focused and lessening the risk to surrounding healthy tissue.

The risks and side effects of withdrawal of testosterone production include; anaemia, impotence, loss of sexual desire, osteoporosis, weight gain, reduced brain function and loss of muscle mass.

As there are many different types of cells in prostate cancer, this may not be suitable for all cases. The more Hormone-sensitive cells are present, the better the response to this treatment.

Although advances are being made with regard to treating prostate cancer, new and varied treatments are emerging as time goes on, it is vital that we do what we can to improve our health and give our immune systems the best chance to overcome illnesses like cancer. We need to give the best chance not only to ourselves but also for those following behind so if you have sons, grandsons or nephews, make sure they know all about the signs for prostate cancer. Don't leave it for them to find out by chance or until it is too late and they have to go through what we are going through now. If you have daughters and nieces, they need to be informed too so that they can pass on the information to their offspring. Prostate cancer is a sex hormone related disease for the most part, similar to breast cancer. Give them this book to read when you have finished with it. It won't all be relevant to them but everything they need to watch out for is in here somewhere.

It is possible for either parent to pass down a predisposition in the genetic trace of the family to either sex children culminating in a potential for developing breast or prostate cancer. This isn't about causing a panic; it is putting younger people in a state of readiness by alerting them to potential health problems in the family line enabling them to monitor changes and take early action if necessary.

If you choose to pass this book onto anyone in your family who is in a vulnerable position with regard to prostate cancer, pointing out the 'symptoms' section just to put them on their guard.

keyhole surgery

Keyhole surgery as it is known, is a fast growing method of minimal invasive therapy, replacing the more invasive therapy procedures that have been carried out previously. It has also proven to be a very effective procedure for many types of medical operations where other methods would be considered too dangerous or time consuming or traumatic for the patient. Using this type of surgery allows hospitalised cases to become day case patients. Recovery time is much shorter and the all round convenience is a very tempting scenario for anyone contemplating surgery.

As with any new process or treatment the positive aspects are focused on more than any negatives. Of course time and money are at the centre of most decision making these days and maybe other considerations are played down at times.

I wasn't offered keyhole surgery, if I had been I might have accepted it. Having gone through the experience I am sure it would have lessened the trauma; with hindsight I am pleased it was not offered.

Most prostate cancers are adenocarcinomas and they occur in the peripheral zone of the prostate as opposed to BPH, which starts in the central zone.

For the best chance of a successful prostatectomy it is vital that tissue surrounding the prostate is also removed, hence the removal of adjacent nerves, as cancer cells could have migrated through the prostate capsule.

No matter what the advantages may be in other respects such as saved time and money, my thoughts are that however skilled the surgeon, working with restricted access rather than with unobstructed access increases the probability of leaving behind a few cells of cancer, but that is my view.

ERECTION SECTION

'Laughter, the most civilized music in the world'
PETER USTINOV

ERECTILE dysfunction and impotence are terms that are often used to describe the same thing but they do have different meanings. Impotence means that your penis is unable to stay erect at all or long enough to complete sexual intercourse. Erectile dysfunction means anything to do with erection problems including impotence.

After prostate treatment of any sort, sexual ability is likely to be affected. Depending on the type of treatment you have had, you may be fortunate in regaining the ability to get an erection naturally mainly if you are younger and had no erection problems before treatment.

If you had a radical prostatectomy, a natural occurring erection is going to be a thing of the past, also if your treatment was less drastic but you had erection problems before, you will be more affected.

Help with this problem is available in various forms the most familiar of which is sildenafil better known as Viagra. Available from your GP in pill form, it works by increasing blood flow into the penis enabling a natural erection to occur. Used by many who have erection problems for a variety of reasons it has become a common remedy although it is less successful when damage to nerve or blood supply vessels is involved.

The next option known as the trade name MUSE is the drug aprostadil, which is a synthetic version of Viagra. It comes in a small plastic applicator, which is used to deposit the drug directly to the site by inserting it down the end of the penis. By rubbing the penis for a few minutes thereby distributing the drug into the tissues, it may serve to produce an erection. If this is not successful for you an even more direct method of delivering the drug to the site is by injection.

This involves using a hypodermic needle to deliver the same drug into the sponge-like tissue that is in either side of your penis. The discomfort is insignificant as the needle is so thin but care needs to be taken to ensure that the needle goes only into the side tissue avoiding obvious veins. Injecting near the top may damage nerves or puncture an artery, near the bottom may penetrate the urethra.

Various strengths are available from ten to forty micrograms. It is wise to start with the lowest and move up in strength as having too high a dose for your need can result in a priapism, an erection that won't subside. This may sound to be desirable but is extremely painful; if it hasn't subsided after three hours try applying lots of ice to the area, if that doesn't work seek medical help.

If you have lost both erectile nerves along with your prostate or the previous applications are ineffective the last option is a vacuum pump. This is a plastic tube with a manual pump on one end and an elasticised rubber ring that fits over the other end.

Placing the tube over the penis and down to the pubic bone then drawing air out by operating the pump creates a vacuum in the tube. This causes blood to flow into your penis producing an erection; the rubber ring is slipped off the tube to fit tightly around the base of your penis trapping the blood. Removing the tube leaves the erection intact, it is advisable to remove the ring after half an hour at most.

Of these options the vacuum pump is obviously the most cumbersome process. It entails using gel to slide the rubber ring onto the tube and to seal around the rubber ring and your skin. The tube also requires gel inside to allow your penis to slide as it forms. Sugar based gels are messy to use as they soon become sticky, making an awkward process more undesirable.

Although the pump ought not to get wet, if you are careful you can forget the gel and do the application in a hot bath. By submerging the penis and the lower part of the tube under the water, the pumping process is easier plus the warmth of the water helps with the process and is more accommodating.

All of the previous mechanical ways of obtaining an erection take away the enjoyment of spontaneity and because of the preparation and planning required, for some the eagerness does subside.

There are other means to obtaining an erection but they involve invasive action, inserting bendable rods into the penis and the like. Anyone considering that sort of action should see a specialist to get all of the details first-hand.

GOOD COMPANY

'life is the vehicle which carries your intentions'
ROGER KENLEY DAWSON

PUTTING prostate cancer into a perspective with other areas of life will for some shed light on the realities of illness and remove the temptation to think that we are alone with our feelings. While it is little consolation to know that others are affected in a similar way, it at least lets us see that others are as real as we are to ourselves.

Stirling Moss, whose name we are all familiar with, has had prostate cancer for a considerable time. He takes good care of himself and is doing very well. Film actor Robert De Niro has prostate cancer as does Roger Moore, also known as The Saint and James Bond.

The American war veteran Colin Powell, film actor Charlton Heston and even Nelson Mandela all have the same condition. Yes you might say, Bob Monkhouse died from it, yes he did but he was seventy-five years old, Harry Secombe died from it too and he was eighty-nine. We must face up to the fact that we have to die of something. Once we accept that fact of life, we are winning.

It was Bob Monkhouse who said 'Dying is an unwritten guarantee that comes with your birth certificate' He accepted his condition and did the best for himself for the time he had left, a lesson we can all learn from.

It isn't about dying though is it, look at Arnold Palmer, he was diagnosed in 1997, Harry Belafonte in 1996 and still touring. Rudy Giuliani Mayor of New York, he was diagnosed in 2000 and is running for the presidency of United States seven years later.

The fact still remains that you are much more likely to die from something else while having prostate cancer, than from it.

MANS BEST FRIEND

'change is not made without inconvenience, even from worse to better'
SAMUEL JOHNSON

CHAMBERS English Dictionary gives the meaning of the word 'co-incidence' as 'the occurrence of events simultaneously or consecutively in a striking manner but without any causal connection between them'

Many would say the following is a coincidence. I no longer believe that coincidence occurs in any context. The following for me is a strong indicator that could lead closer to identifying possible triggers for prostate cancer.

Over hundreds of years various types of dog have played an ever-increasing part in peoples lives. From early days, like man, they were natural hunters and as time has gone on they have progressed alongside man, becoming ever more reliant on their keeper for food and shelter.

In the UK today any dog that is not obviously belonging to someone is rounded up and taken into a safe haven. The neglect of any pet is an offence but dogs in particular are given extra attention as they are regarded more as family members or at least are a central part of mans life.

Even though monkeys are said to be our forebears and pigs are deemed to have close genetic links to humans, we have befriended dogs. There has been a co-dependency build up over centuries.

Monkeys, the commonly accepted branch of ancestry for human beings, do not have prostate cancer.

Our genetic cousins, pigs, which are the cleanest and most intelligent farm animal, do not have prostate cancer.

The only two creatures on Earth with the ability to spontaneously produce prostate cancer are Man and his nearest and dearest domesticated animal friend, the Dog.

Genetically speaking dog is some distance from man with other species in between. How strange it is that none of the species in between are affected with prostate cancer.

Is this another link to confirm that environment and lifestyle are responsible for prostate cancer. Are factors common to both man and dog acting as triggers. Yes I know about family links increasing the likelihood of prostate cancers developing but that doesn't mean the cause is in the genes, it just highlights a predisposition as I have mentioned previously.

Scientific papers report that dogs are capable of developing prostate cancer spontaneously or 'out of the blue' with no mention that there could ever be a connection with environmental factors or issues to do with prepared food. If there is no connection it is worth asking why the only evidence of prostate cancer cells in wolves, the dogs ancestor, is in those living near farmland.

The dog is the closest animal to man with regard to living environment and conditions, we share our houses and the food they eat is processed in the same way as our foodstuffs. Many owners treat them as one of the family.

We know that dogs have prostate cancer now but as there is no evidence of any relative or ancestral species developing it outside of the influence of man it begs the question ' when did the susceptibility begin?'

There simply cannot be an answer to this that discounts all of the subject matter in the following sections. Is there some importance to this that is being disregarded? I certainly think it enlivens the debate about where causes are likely to be found.

Perhaps there is a connection and maybe more and closer attention should be levelled at the wider picture of the Dog prostate problem.

PART TWO

WHAT CAN WE DO?

'If I do what I know I shouldn't, how comes I do what I thought I couldn't'
ROGER KENLEY DAWSON

WELL, when you consider what your Consultant may have said to you there isn't it seems, very much you can do.

LETS START THIS SECTION AGAIN

Just remember that your Consultant is looking at your condition from the outside in, and what he is really saying is that there isn't much more that HE can do about it?

To every event there are different points of view and we are able to stand back from any situation and realise that can choose an alternative point of view or to put it another way, we can adopt a different approach to whatever we are thinking about.

It could well be that there isn't much your Consultant can do but does that mean there is nothing that anyone can do, including you? Of course it doesn't. Let us look at the recent history of prostate cancer again just to see what factors may be influencing the increases of the condition. Finding causes or contributing factors will enable us to make decisions to exclude these from our lives and help us to maintain our future.

If we look at the increase in cases of cancer over the last twenty-five years and particularly prostate cancer, we see that a portion of the increase is due to better detection with PSA testing and screening programmes. When PSA testing became widespread in Europe around 1990 the numbers of recorded cases shot up over the following six to seven years. That was a period of discovering what a more accurate picture was with regard to prostate cancer. When we take that explainable section out of the records, we see clearly that other factors are causing the continuous rise in the number of cases. Without doubt we are collectively contributing to the problem by our lifestyle or some aspect of it.

If we are causing this to happen we need to look at how we are living, what we are eating and drinking and how our food is being prepared. Having done that, our duty to ourselves and others is to remove anything we feel may have been contributing to it, thereby allowing our immune system to come to full strength and do as much as it can of what it is designed to do.

Lets start by looking at what is happening around us that previously we may have given little or no thought to. After doing this we will begin to acknowledge that it is within our power to change things within and for ourselves, we begin to see the world differently to the way we have come to accept.

The first thing to understand is, what and where you are today is the sum total of decisions you have made previously. You may say that others decisions have affected you and that may be so, but how their decisions affect you is up to you. Many people arrive at their present point in life and time mainly by default, often not even realising that they have made the decisions that have brought them to today.. The reality is that your thoughts and emotions have fed your decision making process, which have brought about the actions that have created your present circumstances. There are aspects to your life that maybe you have had little control over, and these you may say have had an effect on your life. Yes but even so, the truth is that you have allowed those aspects to affect your decision-making either consciously or unconsciously, which in turn has brought you to now.

You may be thinking at this point 'what is this to do with my prostate cancer I didn't decide to have prostate cancer'. If you are thinking something like this, it is important to know the following;

The very first process of cancer starts many times everyday in everyone's body, fortunately our very effective immune system is in place to take out rogue processes as soon as they start. Over generations our physical body will adapt to changes we create or accept, in our environment in the way we live, what foods we eat and water we drink.

If we allow changes to be foisted onto our bodies at a rate faster than our bodies can adapt to, or cope with, it is really our immune systems that we are putting under strain. Anything working under stress or constant strain will weaken and become less effective, and so it is with our immune system.

Looking back over the last twenty-five years we see major changes to our environments and foodstuffs; such major changes over a short time are constantly in collision with our physical ability to deal with them. It is little wonder then that cancers of all types are on the increase, particularly digestive tract cancers and hormonal cancers of which many prostate cancers are.

We as a society have come to accept that the way to deal with illness is to go to the GP and receive treatment in the form of pills, potions and invasive action. There is nothing wrong with that but what is sad is that for a large part we have forgotten our response-ability to ourselves to avoid becoming ill in the first place. This complacency, adopted as a society, is our failing.

Prostate cancers as well as other cancers are mainly a disease of an affluent or complacent society and the repercussions are now starting to be felt. Childhood cancers are increasing at a rate not seen before but it isn't something the children have done that causes their illness, it is what we the adults in society are allowing to happen that is contributing to the causes. We aren't choosing to have the cancers directly but we are allowing the changes and by default are contributing to the causes.

The numbers of men diagnosed with prostate cancer has been increasing dramatically over the last fifteen years and the age group of men affected is becoming younger as time goes on.

Even though the official medical chain of command has this information, little is done by way of prevention. The stock response is to provide reactive treatment for the disease as opposed to giving information regarding prevention and educating young males to cut back the overload on immune systems. The ongoing reactive approach to illness is similar to other social ills where managing the problem is preferential to finding solutions that don't cost money.

The Government of the day is choosing to put money to the problem because it is becoming huge, prostate cancer now affects ten per cent of the male population. It is a short term answer, which is the order of the day but a solution will never be found without a change in attitude towards illness. Education at school age with regard to good health is vital if individuals are to accept lifestyles that include preventative aspects.

A large chunk of current day thinking is that we can do what we like with our lives and when we get a problem, someone else will sort it out for us and that is our right. This abdication of response-ability is rife and is storing up huge problems for our young ones for when they become older.

We have to understand that whatever we do for and to ourselves is what we choose to do. We can choose to do nothing at all for ourselves if we wish. Choosing to do nothing is a valid and acceptable decision for those making it, as long as judgement is made using all the relevant information.

Choosing to make the best of our lives is an alternative decision; this of course means different things to different people. One choice might be to do less of what we aren't keen on and go on lots of holidays and just live out the rest of life and take it as it comes. Another choice might be to change the way we have been living and start to pure up our lives to a better standard. Acknowledging that this life is a privilege and for it to continue beneficially for all who are in it requires collective respect and response-ability to and for each other and to life itself. This choice will also bring extra from life when we are more watchful of what we put into it; we shall find a worth more valuable to us. We shall be healthier and in better shape physically and mentally to enjoy every day.

What are we doing to ourselves that lowers the expectation of a longer and healthier life? In your case it may be one thing or a mixture of things and I suspect that as there are various types of prostate cancer cells, it must follow that there are a range of triggers.

Before deciding on any actions, let us look at some of the things in our midst that are known to detrimentally affect health. These are not the only means by which our bodily processes are disrupted but do present a starting point from which we can consider our options.

'If we wish to improve our health, any changes that are genuine, achievable and practical alternatives within our daily lives that achieve this, are worth the effort it takes to implement them.'

Any of the following topics may or may not be factors to do with prostate cancer directly but what is certain is that our immune system which is our ultimate protection is being bombarded with the effects of these and our health threatened in various ways, what is more this is known to be so.

Lets us look at items that we are all familiar with.

I mentioned briefly microwave ovens. The chances are that you have one in your kitchen and it is used on a daily basis like ours was until I started doing my research into prostate cancer. When I discovered how they work and what actually takes place in order for food to be heated, I took ours to the local amenity site.

No doubt you will recall the dark days of the USSR with the continuous flow of awful news that was relayed on our TV screens.

As bad as Russia might have been in many respects, on the grounds of public health and safety they were ahead of where we are today by actually banning the use of microwave ovens in 1976.

Here over thirty years later they are sold daily, for a few pounds without any warnings of the damage that radiation is doing to the food heated in them and consequently to our health.

A more accurate title for a microwave oven is a radiation oven, less attractive I know but would you have bought one with that name, I don't think I would.

Fact: All radiation made by man kills life eventually. Radiation emitted by the sun is not the same, that doesn't cause heat to be generated by friction.

When food is radiated in one of these ovens, the water molecules in the food are agitated with such force that friction from the vibration causes heat, which cooks, warms or thaws your food.

Looking more closely at this process we see that the water molecules are agitated to such a degree that the poles on each molecule are alternated millions of times a second, some say billions; this aggressive action destroys the extremely delicate construction of molecules, they are torn apart and destroyed. The adjacent food molecules are then also deformed or torn apart. This microscopic environment of molecules is transformed immediately into a mix of unnatural cancer causing chemicals, which we then put into our body. Our immune system is put on full alert simply unable to recognise these alien compounds.

Experiments by the Russians using extremely sensitive equipment showed that humans do not even need to eat the food in order to be harmed by it. The exposure to the energy field from the food is enough to cause such changes in the biological balances of the human body that 'microwave' ovens were banned from use throughout Russia in 1976.

The only warnings given regarding safety of 'microwave' ovens is with regard to ill fitting doors causing leaks, not using metal objects, and babies bottles exploding. Nothing is mentioned from the reams of evidence showing that harmful changes occur in all foodstuffs heated with manufactured radiation.

Dr Lita Lee of Hawaii reported as long ago as December 1989 in the Lancet: 'Its bad enough that many babies are not nursed, but now they are given fake milk (dried milk) made even more toxic by microwaving'

If you have owned a microwave radiation oven for years and are thinking that you are all right so it must be ok, well that oven may well have contributed to the weakening of your immune system. As you age and need your immune system even more, the constant onslaught of those toxins will make it less effective.

When we first read of things we use being described as a threat to our health we are naturally sceptical and it takes some thinking about before we feel comfortable with the new suggestion. Well this may be the first you have heard of it but this isn't a new suggestion; the knowledge has been around for years.

'A new idea is first condemned as ridiculous and then dismissed as trivial, until finally, it becomes what everybody knows'
---WILLIAM JAMES

In 1991 Mrs Norma Levitt an American lady, went into hospital for a hip replacement. All went well with her operation until she needed a blood transfusion. The Nurse responsible heated the blood to the correct temperature in a microwave oven instead of the usual method. The blood was given to Norma and she promptly died.

Radiating the blood in a microwave oven created chemical changes transforming the blood into a toxic mix and it poisoned her.

Blood samples taken from humans within fifteen minutes of them having eaten microwaved foods is found to have substantial degenerative characteristics. Experiments have shown that in these tests, white blood cells have become temporarily greatly reduced. White blood cells are a variety of types of cells but are mainly concerned with immunity against infection and cancer. In the above experiment the lack of white cells in samples taken from the limbs might well indicate that they have migrated to the stomach area to deal with the toxic substance recently ingested. Other changes in the blood are shown to be similar to changes known to occur in other precancerous blood samples.

There is some argument relating to microwave radiation and irradiation as used for treatment in radiotherapy and sterilising instruments. Those who believe that microwave radiation is safe argue that each of the two processes use different wavelengths of radiation.

My view is, we know microwaves kill life as it is now being suggested to microwave our dishcloth instead of washing it.

Microwaves sterilise food the same as they do dishcloths and leave behind dangerous compounds, toxins from dead bacteria and lifeless food.

Remember that fresh food is living; when it is cooked it dies but when cooked in a microwave it is turned into something less pleasant. You may say those responsible for our health wouldn't allow this if it was harmful, well it is quite legal in the UK to irradiate food in order to make it last longer on the supermarket shelves. The food is treated with the same radiation that is used to kill cancer cells. It kills all living organisms that it comes into contact with by destroying the cells of the organism, this cannot happen in isolation from the surrounding cells of foodstuff.

Experiments carried out by eminent scientists show that using microwave ovens to heat food compromises health. Attempts were made to silence these facts in Switzerland some years ago and were successful for a period of time. Can you reason with yourself to accept that if you continue to use a microwave radiation oven, you really are not doing the best for yourself or anyone who comes to visit and eat with you.

Knowing that something you are doing is detrimental to your health and choosing not to change what you do is ok. As long as this is with the knowledge that you are undermining your immune system, so weakening your fight against illness and cancer, whether it is the cancer you may have now or one that hasn't started yet.

If you ask any of the official bodies about safety and health risks regarding microwave ovens, they refer to not heating babies bottles in a microwave oven as they become hotter than they seem and burn the babies mouth, neglecting to mention that digestive tract cancers, anywhere from mouth to anus, are increasing at alarming rates. They will also advise not to boil water to make tea in them as putting a teabag in the water causes it to boil over and may scald the person holding the cup, neglecting to mention the reason for the horrendous taste of the water. When water is boiled by microwave, the water becomes a potent unnatural chemical that our bodies are not equipped to deal with.

Take a very healthy pot plant and water it only with water that has been boiled in a microwave oven and over a few days see the change. I have experimented with six varieties of plants, each have died.

We eat food in order to take energy from the food into our own energy system. Experiments have shown that when food is cooked in a steamer, up to fifteen percent of its vital energy is lost in the process, when cooked in the traditional way in a saucepan up to forty five per cent of its vital energy is lost, when cooked in a microwave oven food loses almost all of its vital energy so much so that it isn't worth eating. It may keep its colour but it has become alien to our body and is overworking our immune system.

The financial interests in the UK are such that no law exists requiring health risks to be attached to these machines at the point of sale. What do you think?

THIS TEXT HAS BEEN REMOVED FOLLOWING ADVICE FROM COUNSEL.
IT IS SOMETIMES DIFFICULT TO TELL THE TRUTH.

THIS TEXT HAS BEEN REMOVED FOLLOWING ADVICE FROM COUNSEL.
IT IS SOMETIMES DIFFICULT TO TELL THE TRUTH.

Water as far as our health is concerned is one of the most neglected aspects of our life. The average adult body contains about 90 pints of water and represents between fifty and sixty-five percent of our physical self. Men have more water as a percentage of body volume than women. Every cell in our body contains water except fat cells. Blood is eighty-three percent water, bones are twenty-two percent water and muscle is seventy-five percent water.

Whether we realise it or not, we rely on a supply of good quality water as a foundation for good health. Our water supply companies are responsible for delivering potable water and engage in removing toxins from the water before it is distributed to the public. There is no water shortage; the amount of water on the Earth is exactly the same as when Earth was formed. Water companies engage in cleansing the supply and in order to achieve that add certain chemicals to the water.

You may be aware of these if your water has occasionally tasted 'metallic' or 'like disinfectant' or 'thick'. This is evidence that whatever is being added deliberately, like aluminium sulphate and chlorine, is not being distributed evenly throughout the supply.

Nitrates from chemical farming practices are not removed from the water and on top of that some water companies are adding a chemical fluoride to the water at the request of local health authorities. The chemical fluoride being added has a higher toxicity rating than lead, is an industrial waste product and is added to our water on the basis that it will prevent tooth decay in children. When applied directly to teeth, natural fluoride has a strengthening and beneficial rebuilding effect on the tooth enamel. When it is consumed and passes into the bloodstream it has the opposite effect, undermining the strength in bones and is known to cause primary bone cancer in boys up to twenty years of age as well as being associated with many chronic health conditions.

On tubes of fluoride toothpaste in America there is a health warning on the tube stating 'if more than a pea size amount of toothpaste is swallowed, the person must attend a poisons centre at the local hospital'.

Boys from the ages of six to ten consuming fluoride are most at risk from developing a primary bone cancer during teenage years. The fluoride is taken up as a mineral by the newly forming bones causing malformation of bone cells. This can develop into osteosarcoma up to the age of age nineteen.

A former Scottish Health Minister has given fluoridation of drinking water unqualified support as has a consultant in dental public health for NHS in Scotland. He has asked for the ability to force Scottish Water to fluoridate the supply when asked to do so by the health boards. These are prominent and well-meaning people who are responding to one particular problem in a very specific section of the community.

I contacted Severn Trent PLC to ask their position with regard to the adding of fluoride to drinking water. They didn't seem to be interested in responding although I did receive a copy of a report that gave figures for amounts of chemicals in the water when tests were carried out. I was advised to contact the NHS East Midlands. I did so and my question to them was:

Would you tell me who is ultimately responsible for adding fluoride to the water? Is it yourselves for the decision to do so or the water company for taking the action?

The reply, which took a month to arrive by email, was as follows:

Responsibility for taking the decision to fluoridate a water supply lies with the Strategic Health Authority (SHA). There are clear processes laid down in the fluoride regulations, which include a public consultation process, prior to the decision being taken.

Water providers must fluoridate when requested to do so by the SHA provided they are appropriately indemnified.

Provided they are appropriately indemnified. This means that it is known that problems are going to be caused, but to what extent is not known. No company can be forced to take a path that will result in lengthy class actions against it at a later date so the Government indemnifies the water companies from the outset.

Article 8 of the Human Rights Act forbids mass medication as no person can be made to take medication against their will but the Government Medicine Control Agency defends the action by saying fluoride is not medicine. Anything being administered in order to cause a change in a bodily process is definitely a medicine, if not, what else is it.

You may think that I have drifted from the core subject of this book. No I haven't.

Industrial solvent residues have been found in biopsies of prostate cancers but more than that I am drawing your attention to the fact that when it comes to matters which may affect your health, be responsible to yourself. No matter who is telling you that something is quite safe, ask yourself why are they telling you that. The answer could be they are serving their specific purpose and usually without paying attention to the wider consequences of their actions but you and yours are on the receiving end.

We have just seen how a Scottish Health Minister and a Consultant Dental Public Health expert can be drawn so easily into tunnel vision, seeing only the benefit for a specific problem without taking into account the wider ecological impact on general biological health.

An alternative to adding fluoride to the drinking water to offset tooth decay in children is to teach children to clean their teeth maybe at nursery or primary school. The saying 'Give a man a fish and you will feed him for a day, teach him to fish and you feed him for life' comes to mind. That must be too much like hard work to organize, spike their drinking water instead. That may help to preserve their teeth but bone cancers, allergic reactions and chemical poisoning are someone else's problem.

99% of fluoridated water is used for purposes other than drinking so hundreds of tons of the stuff goes down the drain polluting the water supply. These added chemicals cause allergies to develop in the wider population who as a result develop subdued immune systems. Livestock, given fluoridated water, fall below standards required in order to be classed as organic and if they aren't, they ought to be.

It is illegal to dump fluoride in the sea but OK to put it in the drinking water.

Anyone wishing to interfere with drinking water would do well to reconsider such a move otherwise the next layer of politicians and the like may decide to overcome Monday morning hangovers by adding aspirin to the drinking water.

Water is a particular sensitive subject because we don't get a choice and the toxins that are added to water by the water companies are extremely difficult to remove. Filters don't do it.

There are many issues surrounding processed food in relation to additives that our body has to deal with. When food is fresh, all is well. When food is processed, all sorts of chemicals might be added to it. Additional colour, taste, longer life and better odour give levels of quality that don't exist naturally and are supplemented in order to increase sales.

All of these impurities have to be dealt with by your body. You may have eaten bread rolls or fresh cooked bread and found yourself dropping to sleep half an hour later. That will have been caused by intolerance, usually of an enhancer that is added to cheap flour.

People generally accept that adding these chemicals is in order 'otherwise they wouldn't be allowed to do it'. Well that isn't true. The rulebook may say that it is ok to add chemicals but who is to say correct amounts are added or what correct amounts are. I know these things are monitored but you have to ask who is doing the monitoring, it may be people who are as interested in the common welfare as the two previously mentioned.

Even if the addition of these chemicals is being monitored correctly, who is to say how much of a particular product you can eat before you are un-intentionally overdosing on the additives. We all vary and what one person might be ok with, another may not.

The truth about transfatty acids or transfats, a zero nutritional value and harmful substance that is added to many foodstuffs, has been hitting the headlines for a few years but some manufacturers are at last responding to public opinion.

Fortunately there is a developing climate of openness with regard to what some manufacturers are doing to our foodstuffs.

The media have carried many stories of bad working practices and re-vealed what happens at the production level to what we are actually eating. As the truth unfolds or is leaked regarding fiddling with our food, people become more discerning; the ensuing pressure in many cases causes such practices to be discontinued.

McDonalds restaurant chain has announced that it no longer uses trans-fat in its production of chips. To my knowledge, they never said that they were using it. You see we just don't know what is being used.

It is tempting for food manufacturers to keep using these so-called en-hancers; because without them their products need to be a better quality otherwise they don't sell. There is no obligation to care for the longer term health of the people the food is sold to, over and above the existing legisla-tion, which is weak with regard to public health. This care less attitude is given a form of credibility and defence by standing under a placard saying 'it's business'. Fortunately the more socially responsible of major retailers are reassuringly more attentive to customer needs.

Due to the fierce competition between the larger retailers, better product and informed choice is becoming more common, the trend will continue and as far as food quality is concerned, the future is brighter.

I could go on and on about rubbish we are putting into our bodies; kippers that have never seen smoke, which is okay but they are not kippers, cider that has never seen an apple, which is ok but it isn't cider, sugar that isn't sugar, flavoured snacks that have only chemical additives to create the flavour, cheap wine that is spiced up with additives, milk that isn't milk. By acknowledging to ourselves that what we eat has immediate and longer-term impacts on our general health, we can move forward in taking responsibility for our well being. Let us not fall into the trap of blaming manufacturers; instead let us choose to be watchful and purchase the better product.

After speaking to many people over the last couple of years about choosing better products most say that packaged products have ingredients printed so small they are almost impossible to read. What a breakthrough for health it would be if all ingredients were printed in a minimum size font of say 12. It is the most important information on the pack and giving it that prominence would say much for the product.

Teeth are something that we all should consider with regard to ongoing good health. Even if you clean your teeth regularly, are you cleaning them properly? One in four people over the age of thirty has the beginnings of gum disease and this is due to people using only a brush and not flossing between teeth. Food lodged between teeth is sitting in an acid environment so deteriorates quickly. It begins working its way down the teeth into the gums. Toxins from gum disease and bad teeth are known to be a cause of heart disease but long before the poisons attack the heart muscle our immune system is constantly occupied with subduing the harmful effects of the poisons on the rest of our body. This is another task that our immune system should not have to be doing, by paying attention and cleaning our teeth properly, we can free up our immune system to deal with other tasks and feel noticeably better in the process.

Whether you like it or not you are what you eat and drink. The cells of your body are being rebuilt on a daily basis from the food and drink that you ingest. Where else are you coming from?

If you want the best of health, a clear mind, more energy and a positive attitude there are many things you can do to bring these things about. We have looked at our environment, foodstuffs, water, and at the way we are advised by some of those who are in positions to lead us.

To some of us, it may all seem to be such a major undertaking that we cannot change things. There is too much to change! How will I know I am doing the right thing! How can I keep up with all of this!

At first there doesn't seem much to believe in does there? But there is. You can, if you choose to, believe in yourself. You have the ability to do the very best for yourself and those who you care about. You can decide to do it all at once or not at all or you can decide to find an in-between point and start to make permanent changes to the way you are living. You can decide to do whatever you feel is necessary to promote the best way to be within yourself from today. You can do, but what will you do?

WHAT WILL <u>YOU</u> DO?

'Yes you can, of course you can, you know you can,
but will you'
ROGER KENLEY DAWSON

THE truth is that you can do so much but any difference to your life is only going to come from what you will do.

Anything you may or may not decide to do will be your judgment and choice.

Physical illness is a manifestation of imbalance of energy; we call it dis-ease or dis-stress. By taking positive action with the intention of becoming as fit and healthy as it is possible to do, we can minimise the effect of our condition.

I want to say that with regard to changing your lifestyle or if you are dealing with other health issues, any changes that you make your mind up to implement, clear them first with your GP.

Anything you may decide to do from here is not intended to replace any medical treatment you may be receiving from elsewhere. It is in addition to medical treatment and is to put you on the best available course of action to increase the capability of your immune system.

Only those who have had a diagnosis of cancer know what effect it has. We don't all respond in exactly the same way but without doubt the psychological impact is not a recommended experience; we don't have words to convey our innermost feelings.

From the moment we are captured with our diagnosis, fear or a closely related emotion is locked into our subconscious.

The knowledge of the cancer and the fear share the same compartment and it becomes impossible to think of the condition without disturbing the emotion.

When we feel fear in other circumstances in life, we create a resistance to it and choose to avoid in the future whatever it was that caused the fear.

When the fear is associated with a disease within our body we cannot avoid it in the future so immediately we have inner conflict.

We have inner conflict about an inner conflict.

To reduce the harm that comes from inner conflict we need to deal with the fear of the condition as soon as we are able.

When you mentally resist something you are giving it life, you are saying 'there it is'

Resistance will not eliminate it and it may also serve to fix it more firmly in place.

Accepting the condition as being present is the answer.

Accepting is not the same as welcoming or surrendering. True acceptance will remove the attached emotion, which will lift the cloud and put you into a more positive frame of mind. A positive frame of mind will empower your immune system; a known fact.

You will recall I mentioned that changing your lifestyle too quickly could make you feel worse than you felt before. In order to maximize the benefit to you, change only at a pace you feel comfortable with and can adapt to. There is no rush but adopt a progressive attitude and hold on to the belief that you can make a difference to the quality and quantity of your life.

Changes you make to your lifestyle are going to affect your partner as well so the first thing to do is to ensure that you are working together towards a better future. If you both follow this course of action you will both be on a path to better health and feel physically and mentally fitter than you do today. It is a recipe for better health, whether you are ill or just tired and lethargic. It isn't a magic spell or potion, it is a reassessment of the values you have acquired and a readjustment of the way you live your day-to-day life.

It does need commitment to begin making changes but as you begin to feel better due to the changes, that is the point at which you need to boost your commitment. For some reason with a number of us, as we start to feel better we sort of celebrate by letting go and drift into old habits. It is complacency really, and it is easy to forget that complacency probably contributed to our developing illness in the first place.

By consuming only good quality food, our body can focus on what it does best and that is digest good wholesome food without the hindrances of toxins. Our immune system will strengthen allowing more efficient delivery of oxygen and vital energy to every part of our body.

If we were starting a DIY job in the house we wouldn't start by making a list of what we don't need in order to do the job, so the way forward is to concentrate on what we do need in order to achieve our ambition.

It is fundamental to the success that you are aiming for, to remember that responsibility for the physical condition of your body lies with your mind. This does not apply to any condition or disability you were born with but your mind does decide what you take into your body, rightly or wrongly, either consciously or unconsciously.

First and foremost we need air to survive, lots of it, and the quality of the air we breathe makes a difference to the way we feel. The way we breathe also makes a difference.

Secondly, to distribute oxygen and other nutrients to where they are needed our body uses water. Water is the major part of our life support mechanism, without it nothing would work. The main content of our body is water and that fact alone tells us that it needs to be as clean and pure as is possible to obtain.

Third, we need to look at the food we are eating. What sort of food is it? Has it had all of the goodness processed out of it? Where has it come from? How long has it been around? Is it in good condition?

Why are we eating it? Do we need the energy we expect to get from this food? Are we eating because we are bored? Do we eat a lot of the same sort of food? Have we drifted into a habit of eating that just repeats day after day?

Are we aware that much of the fresh food we buy has been grown using chemicals and lacks vital minerals that modern farming methods have stripped from the soil. Not only are we not getting the minerals we need, we also battle with the chemicals that have been introduced.

Are we really relating that information to our personal health? If not we should be.

How are we preparing the food we eat? As we have already discovered, using a microwave radiation oven destroys food quality, no matter how good the food is to begin with. Are you prepared to make a change for the better?

Do you buy prepared chilled foods packed full of chemicals and salt? Do you add salt to food? Salt is the biggest cause of stomach cancer worldwide.

Do you buy milk, cheese, yoghurt and meat products knowing that they contain residues of antibiotics and other immune depressant chemicals that are injected into the livestock?

When I began to look at the hidden aspects of my daily intake, it appeared to be an overwhelming challenge to transform my life in order to do the best for myself. However I did begin to make changes and very quickly realised that it wasn't overwhelming. At any time I could have stopped and reverted back to the way life had been previously had I wanted to and knowing that made it easier to carry on. I modified on a gradual basis.

I wanted to do it; no one was making me do it. I had chosen to do the best for myself, why would I then choose not to do the best for myself?

The next section is written in the order that I chose to take. It makes no difference where you begin but for a better future, do begin.

Change your way of life and change your life. Determine a new way to be and know the past will lose its power over you.

Make a decision now that you are going to get back into the natural path of your life and take it in the direction that you know in your heart is the right one. Be strong to make the decisions to do what is right for you and yours in discovering this new beginning and make the best of every day you have.

Striving to do the best for yourself for your highest good at all times is as much as you can do, whatever the outcome. Perfection may not be a realistic expectation but the determination to excel and retrieve your future is an incredible quality that you have, choose to use it.

From now you are no longer a victim of this condition, you are the manager who is going to focus positive attention to this problem and accept responsibility to sort it out to the very best of your ability.

START NOW

FOOD

The easiest and most effective action you can take is to throw away your microwave radiation oven. If it goes against the grain because you have recently replaced it, call on your inner determination.

Don't keep it just in case; throw it out. Make this an irreversible decision. Tell your family what you are doing and why you are doing it. Do this to reinforce your own commitment so when they see how you improve over the coming period they we hope, will do the same.

Replace it with a three-tier steamer.

This transition is taking you from the worst way to prepare food to the best way to prepare food. This one thing will retain as much vital energy in the food after cooking, as is possible to do. Eating raw food, well cleaned is the absolute best you can do.

Steaming gently transforms raw food into a cooked state without causing any damage to the food. The amount of goodness retained with this method is the maximum that can be retained in any known practical cooking method. It is so easy to cook by steaming whether using a metal steamer that sits on the cooker or an electric model. We purchased a Tefal Steam Cuisine from Argos for under £30. It is the most used item in our kitchen. The cooking times for different foods are printed on the machine. The whole meal is cooked at the same time. The food is tasty and you find that you don't need so much to eat because you feel more nourished by food cooked this way. We prefer to eat simple food but there is very little that a steamer cannot cope with; obviously it is no good for roasting meat but as I don't eat anything that has had legs, that doesn't bother me. Fish cooked in the steamer is excellent.

The next best way of cooking food is to boil it, this still doesn't cause any damage to the food but the retention of vital elements within the food is less efficient than steaming. If you must boil food do so just enough to cook it, the longer it is left cooking the lower the retention of goodness in the food.

Roasting and toasting are not the best way to cook food. If the surface of the food that has been exposed to the bare heat is eaten such as with toasted sliced bread and particularly if it is well done, the minute burnt particles are a threat to health. They are cancer causing and should be avoided. If you like toast, eat only lightly toasted bread.

The type and quality of food you choose to buy is extremely important so it is important to plan your shopping expedition. When you are actually doing the shopping is when the decisions are made about what to buy so a good way to establish your new regime is to make a list before you go to the shops, that way the temptation to buy what you have previously bought will be gone.

Keep focused on the motive for doing this; you are beginning to make changes that will benefit your health.

As you form new buying and cooking habits, these changes will become insignificant and life will become more positive, easier and more enjoyable.

You have put yourself back in charge of your life and that is where us men like to be.

Only buy the best food and that doesn't mean the most expensive, it means the best food for your requirements.

Buy food that is as fresh as possible and organic. Now if you happen to be someone who thinks this organic idea is a way of taking more money from you, you are right. But let me tell you what else it is; organically grown food grows of its own volition. It hasn't been sprayed with pesticides nor helped along with fertilisers. It has grown the way it was meant to grow, it may not be perfectly shaped but it contains no poison to damage you, that's how it was meant to be.

Fresh organic vegetables may not be uniform in size but you know they haven't been zapped with radiation to make them last longer; they are how they were meant to be.

The vital energy surrounding organic food, which can be photographed using a special camera, is huge compared with the same foodstuff grown using chemicals. It is this aspect that tells the real story. When you eat organic food, you will eat less and get more energy.

The small energy field around processed food is the reason why those who eat processed food most of the time become obese. Without thinking they keep eating because they are seeking nourishment but the processing of food robs it of the vital energy it naturally contains, so those that eat it never really feel nourished, only heavy.

You may be sceptical about organic food but try it for yourself. Farmers markets are a source of good food and increasingly supermarkets are stocking this good quality produce. If you have difficulty getting fresh organic food the next best thing is frozen organic food. Freezing some types of fresh food, carrots for instance breaks it down making it easier for our body to absorb the vital ingredients.

We use Iceland Frozen Foods for supplies. The food there is clearly marked with what it contains as well as what it doesn't.

Only eat enough food for the energy you require. Eating more that you need is weakening and clogs up the bodily systems. It is better to be hungry than overfed. When hungry your body goes into self-preservation mode. It pays attention to what is most important; more blood is sent to the brain and suddenly you become sharper and can think more clearly. Body repairs will be more efficient, you will rest better when you sleep and awake feeling refreshed.

The best guard dogs are always kept on a tight diet.

It is just as important to temper your enthusiasm, missing meals is counter productive. If the body doesn't get some food on a regular basis a different process occurs, the metabolism slows to preserve energy. Eating just enough three times a day is ideal, keeping times as regular as possible.

Always feeling slightly hungry will accelerate your sense of well-being enormously once you have accepted the slight hunger as the normal way to feel. Don't underestimate the human body; it is a miracle of miracles with regard to organisation, efficiency and effectiveness as well as putting up with the way we treat it. Japanese car production lines can't hold a candle to it.

I have mentioned dairy produce and the residues to be found in them. Cattle are injected for various reasons but some of the hormones and immune depressing chemicals stay present in the milk and meat. We are the only mammals to continue to drink milk after being weaned so as adults, do we need it. I think not. Don't forget that cheese and butter and yoghurt are all made from milk, they look different but are all the same thing. Look at these products and question whether you are taking in too big a share of your total nourishment as dairy produce.

On a World scale, there is a graph showing without any doubt that the country with the highest dairy product consumption has the highest number of prostate cancer cases. Whether this could be due to the saturated fats that dairy produce consists of or linked to hormone residues in the produce from chemicals injected into the cattle is not clear. It could of course be a mixture of the two. It could be indicative of other lifestyle choices that are made in those countries which all have with affluent lifestyles.

I make porridge with water and only eat natural yoghurt. I have orange juice on cereals.

Processed foods need to be picked through carefully. I eat tinned tomatoes and some tinned fish for instance but very little else from a tin. I only eat homemade cakes if at all but organic cakes and biscuits are available to buy if you don't have the time or inclination to cook.

Look at the ingredients on packages and tins, if hydrogenated anything is mentioned, put it down again. You don't need to eat anything that has in it preservatives, colourings or additives of any sort. Go for fresh every time. There are all sorts of things you can add to a chopped salad that will do you the world of good, dried fruit, nuts, olives or any fresh fruit or vegetables that will grate or chop.

Treat yourself to a recipe book for home made soups and one for salads, as you begin to feel better because of what you are doing, your enthusiasm will grow too.

If your digestive system isn't quite up to the mark, try taking probiotic drinks, they aid digestion for many.

If you say things like 'I can't do this or that' change what you say to 'I didn't used to be able to do this or that, but now I can'

If you change what you say you will change what you do.

There is no mystique to any of this; you are just as capable as the next person to change what you do to help yourself. There is no need to become obsessed with food. At the moment you are reading through the various changes that you can choose to make to your life but they don't have to be done all at once. Intend to implement these changes at a pace you feel comfortable with and just keep it in mind that you eat to live, not live to eat.

Enjoy making a plan of action with do by dates and details of changes you are going to make. Draw up a weekly menu and stick to it until you have adjusted. If that is too much at once make up a breakfast menu only or change three days a week to start with.

Don't become paranoid about food either, focus your own mind for your own highest good, endeavour for your own benefit. There is no need to talk about what you are doing if you choose not to, instead wait for the positive comments from friends and family as you start to take on your new attitude and outlook.

WATER

Water as well as being the most important nutrient in your body is the most voluminous ingredient in bodily fluids and so plays the biggest part in distributing oxygen and other nutrients as well as collecting and disposing of waste.

It is your bodies transport system.

Water is vital to every minute process that occurs in your body, from microscopic cell renewal to bowel movement.

Good quality drinking water is the basis of good health; drinking the right quantities as a regular daily habit is known to deal with many health issues. Joints and organs are cushioned by water in surrounding cells; body temperature is also controlled with the use of water. Our eyes and mouth are oiled with water. Our digestive system cannot function without sufficient water. Our internal organs are prevented from damage as water dilutes toxins and speeds up the internal body cleansing processes.

We dispose of water when we exhale, urinate, defecate or perspire; this is replaced by drinking water, fruit juice, milk and soup. Drinks containing caffeine, added sugar or alcohol do not count as water replacement; they cause water loss.

Alcohol strips the body of all vitamins. If you must have any make it absolutely minimal and once a week is plenty. If currently you drink more alcohol than is recommended you may find when progressing with these other changes that alcohol is less desirable, if not, make it so. Contrary to popular belief, alcohol does you no good at all, it is a mind altering substance and contributes nothing to your life. It certainly weakens the immune system so try getting tipsy on healthy atmosphere.

The best daily habit is to drink plenty of fresh clean water. Gradually increase the amount of water you drink daily until you are taking in as much as is comfortable up to two litres a day. If you are on medication for a chronic condition or have a heart condition, seek advice from your GP before doing this. Too much water can be worse than not enough so increase intake only up to two litres per day for an adult.

There is undeniable evidence that increasing fresh water intake on a regular basis has been responsible for eradicating chronic illnesses and conditions for which medication has been prescribed, including some asthmas and diabetes.

At first, it may seem as if you are drinking all of the time but you will be surprised at how quickly changes occur. Energy will flow around your body more freely, you will rest more easily at night as the repair mechanisms that function when you are sleeping will have been oiled; joints will ache less as accumulated body waste will be flushed around your lymph system for disposal. Urine will become clear again as waste liquids become diluted; your kidneys and bladder will be better flushed so no longer under duress.

Digestion will improve, as movement of food through the intestine will be easier and coupled with ample high fibre, constipation will become a thing of the past.

As most people don't drink sufficient water, very few of us feel 100 per cent. We have become used to the way we feel and consider that to be normal. If you are affected with tiredness, dry eyes or mouth, constipation, indigestion, kidney pain, leg ache, dry and saggy skin, headaches, lack of concentration or feeling generally lethargic, all of these can be a symptom of dehydration. If you only drink when you are thirsty, you are keeping yourself short of water. Thirst is a warning sign that your body is short of water; the secret is to keep it topped up and not become thirsty. Constantly being insufficiently hydrated creates an inefficient immune system and can lead to serious medical conditions.

Consuming ample clean water is the kindest act you can do for your body. Knowing that chronic conditions in others have been resolved by increasing water intake tells us we need to take serious notice. Diabetes has in some cases been strongly influenced to improvement, according to reports, by water consumption when coupled with a drop in soft drinks.

Prescription medicine makes drug companies a lot of money, is anyone in the health business likely to advise drinking more water when it is virtually free. There is nothing to be lost by trying the water treatment and much to be gained.

If your tap water is unpleasant to drink or if it contains fluoride (you can find out from your water company) then purchase two-litre bottles from the supermarket. If you haven't taken to drinking plain water in your life and find it heavy or tasteless, try slightly sparkling water, it is lighter and refreshing. I buy Caledonian sparkling water from Sainsbury's. They own the spring where that comes from and the trace presence of fluoride in that water is the harmless mineral in its natural state.

Bottled spring water must be bottled at source and additives may be added. Mineral water is taken from underground and has a higher content of minerals, which will be listed on the label. Mineral water may not have additives added but will be cleaned of dirt and grit.

You may feel that improvements to your health are not possible or sound too good to be true. I don't want to convince you to change your mind but I would ask that if you find it all difficult to believe then just suspend your disbelief until you have tried the changes.

Whether you find it easy or not depends on how much you want the outcome. When you decide to aim for your chosen outcome, nothing will be difficult.

AIR

The air that we breathe is often adulterated with substances we could well do without. This type of pollution is troublesome as we can't see it but often if we concentrate we can smell or taste it.

Let us look at quality first of all. We should do all we can to ensure that as much as possible of the air we breathe is clean. There will be times of the day when the air outside will be cleaner according to where you live. If you live by a busy main road is there anywhere you can walk to in five minutes or so that will take you to a quieter place? If not then perhaps early in the morning before the traffic becomes too busy is the best time. This breathing exercise works better if you are sitting, it can be done standing but if you don't normally exert yourself, make sure you are sitting, at least for the first day or two. Don't overdo it; the secret of achieving success with all of this is to go at a pace that you are comfortable with, but progressive.

It is a good idea to begin this at home in front of an open window if possible, just to get used to the breathing pattern.

It is important that there is no background noise such as radio or TV while you are practicing this exercise.

While sitting, if you are able in front of an open window, preferably in a dining type chair, make yourself comfortable, hold your back straight and balancing your head on your shoulders relax your neck and shoulder muscles. Put your hands in your lap or if more comfortable by your side. Make sure your feet are flat on the floor and take your mind to the soles of your feet where they are meeting the floor; keep your mind there for ten seconds or so.

Now begin to breathe in through your nose, expanding your abdomen as you do. Take about four seconds to breathe in, hold the breath for two seconds and breathe out of your mouth giving about four seconds, wait two seconds before repeating. Repeat continuously, all the time focusing your mind on your breathing, listening to your breathing. Feel the air enter your body, be aware that it is held inside you, feel it leave your body, be aware that there is no air in your lungs. Remember, there are these four stages to this breath and each stage is as important as the others.

Take seven breaths using this method and then let your breathing be normal for you. If you practice this three times a day, you will soon be able to do it without having to do the counting. If you feel able, gradually increase the time between breaths to four seconds.

A good posture while doing this is essential, as is relaxing your neck muscles. Develop a smooth and continuous flow to the breathing and as you become familiar with the rhythm, on the in breath imagine and picture the word 'calm' many times floating in on the breath. On the out breath imagine and picture the word 'tension' leaving your body on the breath. By doing this, your mind will adopt the feeling of calm and dispel the feeling of tension. This will work for you as it did for me. It is likely that you will feel a difference after only one session of doing this and after a few days or sooner, you will begin to notice how calm you are becoming inside. A more settled feeling will surround you and the world may well seem like a different place. If you are honest with yourself and you accept that you are capable of changing the way you think just by changing what you do you may want to change even more. I did.

When you understand that you can change what you think by changing what you do and change what you do by changing what you think, there is nothing you cannot change about yourself.

" any complexity in life is the ego trying to undo the simplicity of reality "
LESTER LEVENSON

IDEAL WEIGHT

Dieting to lose weight is not necessary and unlikely to achieve any degree of lasting success. Finding out your ideal weight from your GP and organising your life to become a person of that weight will be achieved. You might say these are the same thing said differently and to some degree you are correct. The way we approach a challenge will determine the outcome. If you focus on losing weight, you are focusing on where you are now or what weight you are now, you will experience internal resistance to losing the weight. If you start to think about losing weight, you will probably also feel a churning stomach, like a washing machine, that is your resistance rising to the challenge you have set. Focus on your ideal weight only, without thought as to where you are now and your journey will begin. What is important in order to achieve success with this as with anything else is to focus on the desired outcome. It doesn't matter what weight you are now, just find your ideal weight and think about and focus on achieving that.

You know consciously if you are too heavy. Being too heavy puts strain on all of your organs and as it takes more energy to move about, you tend to move about less than you would if you were lighter.

Being too heavy is a burden, it is a good idea to be around a comfortable weight for your height and build.

Adopting the measures we have already gone through, good food cooked properly in sufficient proportions to give you the energy you need, will take you to your ideal weight. Drinking as much water as is comfortable up to two litres per day will make losing weight easier to do; drinking water helps the body to metabolise fat, thereby using it up. Do these things and some gentle exercise as described next and that is all you need do.

EXERCISE

It is important to physically move about as often as possible. The varying pressures we impose on our body with movement act as pumping motions that propel bodily systems. By being inactive our systems become clogged up and toxins build up in our body; aches, pains and illnesses can all come from too little movement.

Exercise also gets rid of testosterone, which is a known cancer-supporting hormone.

This doesn't mean you have to undertake dramatic exercises, but within your own capability walk about meaningfully each day; careful, gentle bending and stretching for a few minutes each day will help as long as you feel comfortable. If you are restricted, move whichever way you can. If your legs don't move do a bit of hand jiving and careful shoulder rolling. Moving our arms and legs helps to keep a good blood supply flowing thereby supporting repair processes.

Take care when beginning exercising. Always build up gently, remember there is no rush. A little and often is the best solution.

Exercise doesn't cure cancer but what it does is help our systems to operate and by doing that it supports our immunity.

The body housekeeping subjects I have covered so far give you the strongest building blocks you require to create the foundations for your future good health. Each of the above changes taken individually will make a substantial improvement to your immune system thereby enabling your own body to be stronger in dealing with the effects of your prostate cancer.

By implementing all of the changes as described above, you are doing your utmost to give your body the best chance to do what it is equipped to do in re-establishing a wholesome condition. This is an excellent opportunity to claim your future and make it the best you can expect to have, why would you want any other?

I implemented all of the above changes and quite quickly. I believed that for me time was of the essence. I probably went overboard on one or two things but I got into shape pretty quickly after my operation.

I monitored everything about myself, all that I had taken for granted before took on a value, a substantial value. I paid attention to me for a change.

It is time for you to pay attention to you. I don't mean you and no-one else, it means putting yourself first without being selfish.

I am very interested in knowing how people are progressing with prostate cancer. If you feel inclined, send me your details and keep me up to date with how you are dealing with it and how you are moving ahead.

If you would like to contact me about any aspects of the above regime, please refer to the back of this book for contact details.

IMMUNE BOOSTERS

Correct nutrition is the key.

The word diet refers here to what is eaten and is nothing to do with slimming.

The effects of a single type of food on the body are greatly influenced by other foods so it is important to eat a balanced and varied diet.

Diet can cause cancer and diet can prevent cancer. So far there is no official proof that diet can cure cancer although there are many who claim the opposite. There are recorded cases of men who had a diagnosis of prostate cancer and by, they say, very strict control of food intake and food value, along with relaxation sessions on a daily basis have become cancer free. There is no reason to doubt these claims; instead we should endeavour to follow in the path of these men.

There maybe no proof that diet can cure cancer but it is certainly known that diet can influence the rate of tumour growth. A poor diet that impairs the immune system will allow tumour growth to develop. Don't forget, your immune system will continue to work at keeping you in good health but it needs all the help it can get.

The following foods are believed to assist your disease-beating programme considerably and should be included in your daily intake.

Garlic is an all round health booster and known to have been so for many years. Scientific studies have shown that garlic neutralises cancer-causing chemicals reducing the rate of tumour growth. Studies have shown that those who eat garlic regularly have much lower cancer rates than those who don't eat garlic.

Onions are deemed to be just as active, mopping up cancer causing agents in the body. They both should be eaten as near to raw as possible. If adding to the cooking, do so two minutes before serving. No onion is recommended above another so all types are effective.

Broccoli, cabbage and Brussels sprouts should be included each day. Experiments have shown that three servings a day will reduce the onset of prostate cancer by 41%. These plants contain chemicals called Indoles that are known to reduce the potency of the hormone oestrogen, which encourages certain cancers to grow. The powerful effects of some plant chemicals not only prevent cancers forming but also slow the growth of cancers.

Mushrooms are an invaluable source of selenium, which is known to lower PSA levels and to inhibit tumour growth.

Shitake mushrooms are celebrated for their health giving qualities in the Far East. Herbalists recommend them for a long and healthy life. Scientists in the West have decided that the reason for their efficacy is they stimulate the immune system. When looking at the reasons why certain foods and chemicals are recommended with regard to good health, over and over again we see reference to their effect on our immune system. By eating to support, strengthen and stimulate our immune system while cutting out that which undermines it, is the very best we can do to achieve our best health.

A study at Harvard Medical School by Dr Edward Giovannucci examined the dietary habits of 47000 male health care professionals. It showed that men who had ten or more servings of tomato product per week were 45% less likely to develop prostate cancer compared with men who had no servings.

Ongoing research into Lycopene is showing that it is active in reinforcing our immune system by inhibiting various types of cancer formation and growth and is particularly active with prostate cancer. Lycopene is the red pigment in fruits particularly concentrated in tomatoes; accessing this is easiest by eating tomato ketchup or puree. Any red vegetable or fruit is a source but tomatoes cooked at high temperature with a little oil is said to release the pigment and enable easier absorption into the body.

Lycopene is also found in pomegranates, watermelon, pink grapefruit, and red peppers. A

Although Lycopene and vitamin D are known anti cancer agents, experiments have proved much enhanced benefit when they are used together.

Fructose found in fruit and honey is a simple sugar, which stimulates the body to create vitamin D, an active nutrient.

Fresh fruit also contains anti oxidants that reinforce the effect of vitamins.

Wholegrain breads and cereals are an essential part of a good diet providing roughage to keep things flowing as well as vital elements in the grains.

Herbs can be used to add flavour to food. If you have no garden area it is easy to create a small garden of herbs on the kitchen windowsill, that way they are as fresh as they can be.

Mineral and vitamin supplements are an option; consider whether taking them at all is the right thing for you to do. Many readily available supplements don't contain the active ingredient in a form that can be easily absorbed by the body. It is far better to acquire vitamins and minerals from foodstuffs. Eating a balanced and varied diet is a more positive way of ensuring your body is correctly vitalized.

Shellfish, nuts and seeds, herring, mackerel and sardines will provide plenty of zinc, which is known to be well below normal levels in the cells of enlarged prostates.

Regular sunlight is a must; notice how you feel better just for being in the fresh air and sunlight. Anything you do that makes you feel better in a wholesome way is boosting your immunity to illness, that is what you are feeling when you say you feel better. Heat and light from the sun boost the immune system but be sensible, too much is worse than not enough.

SLEEP

Probably the most underrated aspect of our life when considering health issues, sleep is something we need to support our life systems and if we don't get the right sort and the right amount we change, don't we. Tiredness becomes irritability, aches and pains set in and eventually we may develop some sort of illness; we certainly become susceptible to cold and flu viruses. The reason for this is our immune system is not getting the body and mind state that it needs, in order to be effective. It can't then keep up with what is required of it and we become vulnerable. On the surface it may be a short term cold but what is happening at a deeper level?

For the immune system to work at its best we need to be in a completely relaxed state, allowing our mental and physical parts to do the repairing processes needed after a day of activity, whatever that entailed.

We spend almost a third of our life in bed and yet most people buy near to the cheapest bed in the shop, reassuring themselves they have done the right thing because they haven't bought the cheapest bed available.

A firm mattress on a solid base will give support to all of the body, reducing sleep tension and provide the ideal platform for good rest. If this doesn't suit you, get as near to it as you can.

Prepare for sleep by not eating or drinking anything for three hours before going to bed and remember that one hour of sleep before midnight is worth two after midnight.

Look forward to the rest you are going to have and if you have trouble going to sleep, you may decide to try this.

Lay in a comfortable position but not on your left side if you can help it, breathe deeply for six or seven times, each time taking four seconds to breathe in and four seconds to breathe out with two seconds between each of those. Then say the word 'off' softly to yourself or out loud if you can, and repeat every five seconds or so while concentrating on the word itself. See the word behind your eyelids, hear the word and focus your mind on the word. If it doesn't work the first time, don't give up on it but don't try too hard either, it will work eventually.

When you wake, get out of bed carefully and progressively and start your day.

If this sounds a boring way to live, make a habit of doing five out of the seven nights or try every other night, any amount of nights per week is going to make a difference. Buy a good bed!

WISE TO LEAVE OUT

By looking carefully at statistics and results of studies carried out we can identify foodstuffs that present the greatest potential risk or affect our ability to deal with prostate cancer. The highest rates in the world of prostate cancer are in the United States and Sweden and these countries have the highest consumption of saturated fats, those being animal and dairy products. The lowest rates of prostate cancer are in China and India where there is the lowest consumption of animal and dairy produce. Either animal fat itself or residue in the fat from injected chemicals may have a link or be a trigger for prostate cancer. It could be that other common factors in these same countries are the causes. Whatever it may be, we need to concentrate on forming our lives in a way that gives us the health we want.

Some fat is needed to enable bodily processes to take place but saturated fat particularly, should for the most part be excluded. It is wise to reduce all fat intakes to a minimal amount.

Reduce to a minimum; red meat, cream, cheese, full milk,

butter, chicken & turkey skin or dark meat, farmed fish unless trimmed of fat, margarines, processed baked goods.

The most effective first step to reducing fat intake is to throw away the frying pan. Irrespective of what type of fat is used for frying, olive oil, vegetable oil or lard, fried food is better off the menu.

I will mention here once more that eggs are not dairy produce; some people seem to think they are but I have checked and cows don't lay eggs.

Processed or baked snacks that list 'partially hydrogenated oil' should be avoided, as should chilled prepared meals.

Salt tries your immune system, use absolute minimum and choose foods that are salt free. If you add salt to bring out the taste of food, try using mustard or pepper or herbs instead but keep away from vinegar.

Salt as well as nitrates occur naturally, it is when they are added either as a salt preservative or nitrate fertiliser that the proportions become excessive. They are used in preserved meats like bacon and ham, which should be reduced to a minimum.

Sugar is another food we add to aid taste. There is ample natural sugars in a balanced diet, avoid adding sugar altogether for maximum progress.

Carrying extra weight puts a further burden on your immune system and for some reason the fat that gathers around the middle produces additional surplus hormones that the body does not need but has to cope with. These hormones are thought to play a part in promoting the processes that cancers originate from.

I have heard it said that a refrigerator is a cupboard where food is stored until it goes green. Keep yours in best of order, ensure it is clean and only contains food that is going to be eaten within four days if possible. Throw old food away; don't keep pushing it to the back. Mould sends out tentacles into the food and is not always visible, so breaking off that which you can see does not get rid of it.

Mould on hard cheese can be trimmed but never on soft cheeses. Ideally do not eat food that has mould on it or food that has been left uncovered next to open mouldy food, the spores travel and may not be visible.

PART THREE

MY PERSONAL EXPERIENCE

'for some, life is a moment by moment business'
ROGER KENLEY DAWSON

WITH all of the dictionaries and thesaurus at my disposal, I would still find it impossible to convey the collection of feelings experienced just after the time of being told that I had cancer cells present in my biopsy tissues. A diagnosis of cancer pulls the rug from under the life of most men and it did so for me.

I felt as if I was heading for the cliff edge and there was nothing I could do about it. Suddenly I had no control over my fate. An invisible enemy was burgling me of my good health from the inside.

What about my wife? What about my family? I won't see my Grandkids grow up. How can I, this person, me, be going to my GP one day with a chest infection and finish up with a diagnosis of prostate cancer.

I remember the physical and mental effect I experienced when told the news. At first it was disbelief, I asked questions as if I was talking about someone else. On the way out of the hospital, I was saying to Vicky my wife, 'it is ok', 'I feel alright', and I did. It was later when the reality was sinking in that the confused feelings started to take effect. Mixed up feelings of anxiety, frustration, despair, in fact just about every emotion I possessed came to the surface except for joy and happiness.

I have discovered ways to deal with the pain and anguish of the days since diagnosis and have no problem in recalling the events, but now without the pain. If you are going through a time like that now, please believe me it will pass, it just takes time.

If you need help with dealing with it, see details in the back of this book.

The emptiness did start to fill again, slowly and differently and it took time but it did fill.

The only way I could see to climb out of the mentally colourless, two dimensional world I had become embedded in was to bring myself to talk about and understand my condition, but how could I, I didn't know anything about it.

I am extremely fortunate to have an understanding wife who put aside her own feelings, at least when I was in earshot, and steered me through the mental trauma.

Together we started to explore the medical world, trying to find sense and reason to this disease that, until then had always been someone else's misfortune to acquire.

Valuing life as we do and not wanting to be in a position where it was ebbing away too quickly or unnecessarily, we gathered knowledge from wherever we could and, dare I say, became experts in about two months. Well that is what we thought at the time.

It was only much later when we realised that all we had studied were the scientific journals and reports, but to become an all round expert on something like this, it needs an understanding of other patient's experiences.

At that time though, the studying and enquiring and questioning helped me to put my situation into perspective and get life back on some sort of even keel. More stormy seas were waiting ahead but for the time being I started to feel in control again. Had I not pursued the desire to understand what was happening to me, I wouldn't have got over this in the way that I have.

I suggest to anyone with a PC or any health condition that a lot of comfort can be gained from knowing and understanding more about the background of your condition than you do now. I do know that some people say they would rather not know, but that feeling is based on fear.

It is overcoming fear, by seeking knowledge about your condition that will help to bring comfort.

For me it all started when I had a chest infection and went to my GP. Dr Pathak MBE. Not having had chest infections or anything similar before, I expected to be rid of it quite quickly with antibiotics. I was very healthy otherwise, active and I thought, fit.

I had my first course of antibiotics, the chest infection cleared up. . . .then came back again. I went back to Dr Pathak who gave me a stronger dose. The infection went. . . .then came back again. I went back to my friendly GP who asked if I had any other symptoms. I had been having a bit of difficulty maintaining erections lately so I volunteered that, it was a bit difficult but that said, Dr Pathak homed straight in on that and asked me to go to the hospital for a blood test. He asked with some urgency if I could go that day, I said I could so he wrote out a form for me to take. I remember thinking how keen he was being but I went straight to the Hospital and had a blood test; that I thought was that.

Three days later, the receptionist at the surgery telephoned me and asked if I could go to the surgery for an appointment the next day. At that time, I was completely unknowing about all that was about to happen. I said I couldn't go the next day but I would be able to go on Monday.

Monday came and I went to the surgery, saw Dr Pathak who explained that the results from my blood test had come back with some urgency and he was making an appointment for me to see a specialist at the Urology Department, City Hospital, Nottingham. He said I might see signs up about cancer but it didn't mean I had cancer, many things can cause the abnormal blood test results but the appointment was just to make sure everything was ok.

Off I went, quite confident that a mistake had been made and all was well.

Ten days later, ultra quick time, I went along to the Urology Department at City Hospital, Nottingham, with my lovely wife and we arrived at the waiting area, which was choc-a-block with people of all ages. I just felt that I didn't belong there for some reason and when it would be discovered that I had inflammation, I wouldn't need to go again.

Two hours waiting saw me in to see Mr. Owen Cole who asked me for a recap of events and suggested that I have another blood test to eradicate any errors. I had a blood test that day and an appointment was made for me for the following week to attend for the result.

23rd March. The following week arrived; still I was convinced that all was well. We went back to the Hospital and the full waiting room, sat for a two-hour wait and saw a different person. He explained that my second blood test had similar results to the first and the next stage was to have a biopsy that would give an accurate picture of what was going on inside my body.

I was to go into the cubicle next door and a nurse with an assistant would talk me through what was required.

OK I said, going along with all of this.

Going into the cubicle I was asked to drop my pants and lay sort of sideways on a bench. There was a lot of equipment in this small room and I remember thinking how big the hospital was and all of this was crammed into this small space.

What was about to happen was; a sonar gun was to be inserted into my bottom and that would create a picture of my prostate gland on a screen, then along with the sonar gun was another instrument that had a hollow needle on the end of it.

The process here was, the operative would use the sonar device to build a picture on the screen then use the picture to direct the gun with the needle to the prostate. The needle gun, when fired would send out the hollow needle and retract it, very quickly removing a plug of tissue from the prostate; this would be repeated about eight times or so in all.

I had an injection to numb the pain from this procedure and to some degree it worked. It was very uncomfortable, there was no enema and trying to overcome the urgency to shit made my eyes bulge.

It was over reasonably quickly. I asked too many questions I think, as there was an irritation in the voice of the replies I was getting. I asked the diameter of the needle and how fast did cancers grow and did my prostate feel ok to him. It was a surreal situation really and most, I think, would have done it all in silence.

One of the needle shots missed its target and felt like a bee sting. I said so and was told that it was only six months previously that the pain killing injections had been introduced. I took this to be a polite way of saying it could be a lot worse.

Each of the shots felt like an elastic band being flicked hard on the inner forearm. That's about as near as I can describe.

I was given some huge tablets to take, very strong antibiotics to combat infection, and told to take it easy with my feet up for four days. If I felt faint or got a high fever, I was to phone three nines.

I drove home saying all was fine, and it was, at least until the local anaesthetic wore off.

I then started to sweat, my legs were shaking, my prostate gland felt like it was a red-hot tennis ball and I didn't feel so good. After three days I went for a walk up the road, about two hundred yards was about as far as I could manage. I was weak and breaking out in waves of sweat. I thought to myself 'why didn't they give me an enema, surely it is asking for infections by not doing so when taking a biopsy through the bowel wall' I then started to wonder whether any cancer cells could have been released into the blood stream by the same route that the infection I was now experiencing, had arrived in the prostate.

This was the beginning of the new era.

8th April. Back once more to the Urology Department. A three hour wait this time, with apologies from the staff. Things do happen and I don't mind waiting, I am thankful to live in a part of the world where these services are available.

So in we go to see Mr. Cole who has my thickening file in front of him. We sit down. 'well, it's as we thought, there are cancer cells present in the prostate'. There really is only one way to say something like that to someone and that is to say it. Secretly I had come to expect the worst-case scenario as a safety mechanism; think the worst and you won't be disappointed.

What I did notice was my wife's jaw drop. The first time in my life I had seen anyone's jaw drop. I had heard the expression but never witnessed it until that day.

I maintained my composure with some ease really; I am quite good at that. The worse the situation, the stronger I become, in the short term. I asked what the Gleason scale was (see the chapter) and after he acknowledged that I must have been doing some homework, he said six. I asked him what the prognosis was and he said he would talk us through the various options for available treatment, we could go away and think about it and let him know.

One of the options was to have an operation, not everyone gets that option. I nearly didn't. My PSA level was 16.5 (normal is about 4) Mr. Cole said 'if it had been 20, I wouldn't operate'. I assume from that, the cancer at a reading of 20 is likely to have broken through the gland wall and set up home elsewhere making it pointless operating. Once these things are on the move, the outlook has a potential to change differently.

The operation being offered was a radical prostatectomy. This is the complete removal of the prostate gland and surrounding tissue.

Radiotherapy was another option but I could go and talk to the Radiotherapist to get the information on that.

Another option was to do nothing. I asked what the outcome would be if I did nothing. He said I would begin to get problems within two years and it would require some attention within that time.

We were to go away and think about what we wanted to do. How long do I have to make a decision? 'Don't leave it too long' how long is too long? 'No more than six weeks'

Off home we went. This time it was different going home. Vicky asked me if I was all right as we came out of the hospital, she probably asked because up to then, there had not been any reaction. She was probably thinking it was the calm before the storm. It was.

Made it home full of distress. Physically shaken to the core, floating yet sinking.

The following days were horrendous. Life became like a dream. Suddenly I have cancer, you know, that killer disease that people get. Not only am I watching this real world picture, I am in it too. My immortality had evaporated.

The next day, I got up in the morning, shed tears in disbelief, then sat on the sofa all day and said not a word. The world had stopped. Totally preoccupied with disbelief and cancer over the next day or two, my head became full of the thoughts of cancer, with my imagination playing overtime. Disbelief started to become fear, and all the things that cancer could do to me became loud and violent in my head. It could kill me. It could cause me to live the rest of my life in violent agony.

I could lose my dignity and have to rely on others for everything. Oh, the emotion with those thoughts.

The fear became a mixture of disbelief, fear and anxiety.

I became a stranger to myself; a void set in followed by the start of a bout of depression. I have heard the expression 'being beside yourself' and from then I knew what it meant. It was as if my soul had slipped out of my body to get away from the reality and I was standing at the side of me.

It was a fair few days before I started to get things in perspective again. Goodness knows what that time was like for the best person in my life, my soul mate. She put up with an awful lot at that time.

I gathered my wits eventually and decided that as I had this dread disease, I would deal with things as they should be dealt with. I decided to arrange my funeral.

I contacted the funeral directors that I wanted to use and asked them to send me an information pack. I sorted out the service and all of the trimmings. I wrote letters to each member of my family, to be distributed after my demise.

I told our adult children that I was on my way out, then having paid attention to the things I wouldn't want to leave for others to sort out, set about trying to make it not so.

What could I do to remove this rogue process?

Sitting down with pen and paper, we made a list of all of the things that we knew we could do, after which we made a list of what we thought we could do. We decided to look at alternative treatments, see what was on offer, enquire and get as much information as we could about them.

We went to see a Homeopath who was recommended to me. She had treated cancer patients over a period of twenty-five years or so and had very good results. We travelled to Manchester and had a meeting with the lady who was very pleasant and took her time evaluating my position. While I was talking to her, it suddenly hit me again that I was talking about myself and tears flowed. When it started like that, it just came from nowhere. She said; to her mind, the best course of action was to have the operation and use homeopathy as a supportive treatment.

She also suggested counselling might be helpful. My tears were born out of frustration more than anything else. I didn't go for any counselling.

We next went to see the Radiotherapist at the hospital to get the facts from him with regard to what he could do for me.

That was interesting. Having a chat with him was quite sobering. I had thought that it was good to have the choice of either an operation or Radiotherapy, 'different today, nobody telling you what to do, there's a choice'.

He explained that the reason the choice between operation and radiography is available, is that statistics show one course of action to be no better than the other, so down to personal choice it is.

With the treatment he was offering, there were no guarantees. He was quite open and straight with the information he was giving. No matter how carefully the process is performed, there is the potential for damage to the surrounding tissue. Damage to the surrounding tissue could be damage to the bowel or bladder, causing anything from irritation to incontinence, from temporary to permanent.

Irritation could mean bleeding, secretions, constipation, diarrhoea, or a feeling of urgency to use the toilet. Incontinence means nappies or a bottle strapped to the shin with a tube going to the penis.

Permanent means forever.

Even with all of these potential after effects there was no guarantee of eradicating the cancer.

The thought of all these potential negative aspects was to say the least, off-putting.

Over recent times, good records have been kept of the various stages of diagnosis, the treatments that followed and the eventual outcomes. This enables with a margin of error, an outcome to be assessed based on previous experience.

I say margin of error because the exact comparison of one case to another doesn't really exist. We are all different to some degree and it is that degree which is the unknown quantity.

I asked the Radiotherapist, knowing what he does about outcomes and the rest, what he would do if he were in my shoes. He said if I were in your shoes, I would have the operation. I asked him why he would choose the operation when he is a Radiotherapist. He said because if you have the operation first and it isn't successful, you can then have the Radiotherapy, but if you have the Radiotherapy first and it doesn't work, you can't have the operation after. Scar tissue won't allow.

That was good enough for me.

After dismissing various other alternatives, Chinese formulas, American wonder drugs, diets and dream potions,

I telephoned the Hospital to say yes to the operation.

There are other options for treatment. I wasn't offered any at the time but I looked into all that was available and didn't fancy any of them. Each one seemed to me to be more risky than complete removal. Killing off the rogue cells by radiation or freezing but leaving them in place, or removing by keyhole surgery just didn't feel thorough enough to me. (see treatment chapter)

My first appointment after that point was with a nurse called Chris. He was a very thorough person and his job was to talk me through the whole procedure from start to finish.

As Chris described the course of action from then on, it became clear that for the period leading up to going into the operating theatre, everything was described as fact. For the period after the operation, most of the outcome was described as expectation. This drove home the reality of where I was and where I might be going.

It was of course how it had to be. There are no guarantees with any of this, only expectation based on the records of what had gone before.

The odds were favourable. I had confidence in the people who were responsible for the procedures. I was happy to continue and did so.

I went to the next room to be weighed. I wasn't overweight as I have always been quite fit and agile, so I was ok weight-wise. The next stop was for an ECG (heart fitness measurement). My heart was deemed ok. Blood pressure was ok. After these preliminary tests, I was sent for an MRI scan and a bone scan.

It would be dependent on these coming out ok that the operation could go ahead. The reason for these scans was to determine whether the cancer could be traced to anywhere else in my body. If it could, the operation was not available.

The MRI scan was strange to say the least. The machine was in a room of it's own with one operator. Quite a size really, this machine with daunting looks about it. Having been asked to remove any metal wares I may have about my person, and after assuring the operator I hadn't any metal implants, I laid on a flatbed at the opening of a short tunnel. I was told it was ok to have someone to sit with me should claustrophobia be a problem for me. I was feeling delicate at that time so my faithful sat at the machine with me. On this machine, I moved through the tunnel from head to toe, very slowly.

For those of you who remember Quatermass and the Pit, that is what the experience reminded me of, mostly by the noise of the machine. The noise the machine emitted was said to be like a woodpecker but if I heard a woodpecker making that noise, I just might go indoors.

That lasted for quite a time, about forty minutes or so.

There were no physical effects.

On another day I went along for a bone scan. Before going in for this scan, I was injected with a mild radioactive substance, which would apparently distribute itself all over my body and I was assured there would be no noticeable effects. I did wonder about that at one point though and that was when I noticed a toilet that was only to be used by those who had this injection, apparently it isn't good practice to put radioactive urine into the main sewer, so it went elsewhere.

I was to wait about an hour for this substance to distribute around my body, and then went in for the scan.

The scanner was a similar but much smaller design to the previous scanner. In this case I was stationary and the scanner moved over me. I was told to keep very still and this took half an hour or so. With this scan, I had to wait in the waiting room for the results. After about ten minutes, I was escorted to the x-ray department to have what became four x-rays on my left ribcage. When I asked why this was I was told that my lungs were being checked.

Apparently the bone scan picks up any metabolic activity that is exceptional, it could be where cancer is active, but it could also be arthritis or a recent fracture.

Eventually, we went home. Tired but things were going ok so far.

A further appointment with Mr. Cole verified that the scans and x-rays were clear and we could plan for the operation.

I opted for Monday June 7. For the next few weeks, I concentrated on getting as fit as I could without overdoing it. I ate properly, left off alcohol, went for brisk walks and generally kept to an early night schedule. As well as getting into shape physically, I was psyching myself up with all of this really.

I went along to the Hospital on the Sunday, arriving at about lunchtime as directed, was admitted and allocated a bed. That evening I had a visit from a nurse who was just managing to speak the language. She was checking the paperwork, next of kin, and 'sign this please'.

I was told that I would be going down for surgery at about half past eight in the morning. I went to sleep about ten o'clock.

At five o'clock after a patchy nights sleep, I was wide-awake. There was activity all around most of the night so really it was a bit like sleeping in the daytime. I reminded myself that it wasn't a hotel and that the staff duties continue around the clock.

I got up and had a shower and a cup of tea at 5.45, the latest I could have a drink was up to six o'clock.

Chatting to one or two more who were also having treatment that day, the feelings of anxiety weren't too far away, either in those I was chatting to or myself, but the decision had been made and it was going to happen.

It was Monday morning and I was going down for surgery quite soon and was now looking forward to getting it all over with. At seven o'clock I was asked if I was feeling ok and would I like a sedative. I remember thinking to myself what a thoughtful gesture, it was reassuring in a way to know that in spite of all that is being done for me, time is made for that thought. I declined but felt better just for being asked. When mentioning my thoughts to a fellow patient, he said 'well, its only a pill'. He was right of course but for me it represented much more.

Two anaesthetists paid me a visit and talked briefly through what was to happen. I signed more papers and off they went saying they would see me later.

Walking to the operating theatre wasn't allowed, so I was installed on a trolley and pushed. Corridors, lift, corridor, double doors then equipment and five people all in gowns.

I was put immediately at ease with all of them. They introduced themselves to me as they were preparing things.

The procedure was explained to me and I was easy with this team.

I was to have an epidural, a spinal injection that would numb all pain below the waistline, and a general anaesthetic; having the two allows the general anaesthetic to be weaker. I liked that idea, thinking to myself that 'someone's thought this through' although I hadn't had any thoughts to the contrary, it just was that the whole process seemed so well organized, it had a natural flow sort of feeling to it. If you think some of these thoughts are a little peculiar, just remember where I was while I was doing the thinking.

Adopting a curled position, I had a painless injection in my spine, followed by quite a large injection through some plastic ware that had been installed in the back of my hand. I remember saying how calm I was feeling as this liquid was ballooning my hand. Then nothing.

I awoke from blackness and a dreamless state in a recovery room. The nurse asked me my name and remarkably I could remember. I couldn't remember much else and it took some time to remember what I was doing there. I had no pain or discomfort. I was told not to lift my head off the pillow otherwise I would develop a headache due to the anaesthetic. After what seemed longer but was probably a couple of hours, I was taken back to the ward and allocated one of four beds at one end of the ward along with three other people. This was the high dependency section of the ward.

I had drain tubes from either side of my abdomen that went into plastic vacuum bottles and a catheter in my penis, draining to another plastic bottle, a liquid drip that I am not too sure about and another drip containing morphine.

I had no pain or discomfort. The pain control was amazing.

I felt quite ok when I was fully back in this world.

I was having my blood pressure and temperature taken every hour and attention was paid to every detail.

I had had fitted tight long white socks which were to combat blood clots forming in the legs. The likelihood of this happening, increases after an operation and more so with staying in bed for extended periods.

The most peculiar thing I can remember experiencing in my life happened over the next forty-eight hours. My family came to see me and I was managing to sit up in bed probably looking like and certainly feeling like plastic 'Robocop'. As I was talking to my visitors, I periodically closed my eyes for a few seconds. When I did this I was in a different place amongst different people.

I couldn't believe this, just by closing my eyes I was transported to elsewhere. These other people were just as real as those around my bed, in colour and chatting away.

When later that day I mentioned to one of the nurses that strange things had been happening in my head, (I wasn't too specific in case I might be carted off) she said 'yes, that will be the morphine' I said, is it? She said 'yes, what do you think the druggies want to get hold of it for'

I had not given such a thing any thought before and decided that I wouldn't want that voluntarily at any time.

When I asked a fellow patient whether he had had any strange experience, he said no but had heard that the week before someone had got out of his bed and ran down the corridor because someone was coming up out of the floor to stab him. I don't know whether the tale was true or not but I thought no more about it.

On the Tuesday night it was thirty-three degrees in the hospital and very uncomfortable. I couldn't sleep; I was wet through and restless. Shuffling about in the bed I noticed that the dressing from my back had come off and there was an unusual feeling in my thighs. It was about two o'clock in the morning, I rang for the nurse who came along and said I had lost the tube that had been inserted in my back that had been delivering the morphine. She said we had better get someone pretty quick before the morphine wears off. I said can't you put it back? No she said. Off she went. Five minutes later along came an anaesthetist who rigged up a morphine bottle on a stand operated by a small hand held pump.

It's a good job we got that sorted for you, he said, if the morphine had worn off you would have been in agony. Thank goodness for that. I thought.

In some ways, the week went quite quickly and in other ways it dragged. The staff were attentive and things were done on a regular basis. Everything looked to be organized.

I had a ten-inch cut from my pubic bone to my navel, which was clipped with metal staples and was a bit sore. I was having several pills four or so times a day to deal with pain and other things, and even a pill to counter any adverse effects from other pills.

The food was good, the tea was good, and the people were pleasant. I remember wondering what all the complaining was about that had been reported in the press over the years. Regular samples of blood were taken to test oxygen levels. The medical men came round every day to check that all was well. Blood pressure and temperature was taken several times a day.

On Wednesday evening the morphine disappeared and I went onto tablets for pain. The vacuum drains that were in either side of my abdomen were removed on Thursday. That was a most peculiar feeling, which is very difficult to put into words, not painful but sort of, no, I can't explain it.

All went straightforwardly until Thursday. I had become aware of a strange smell and told the nurse who was to be changing my dressing. She looked at my wound and said it was ok. I had my dressing changed and just after lunchtime, which was about four hours later, the smell had become very strong to me. I told the nurse who decided to have another look at my wound. When she had removed the dressing, it was now obviously infected. It had all happened within a few hours. What intrigued me about it was the fact that I could smell the infection from the inside and it didn't smell from the outside. I was told that this form of self-awareness is not uncommon.

The infection seemed to have come from nowhere. Several of the metal clips were removed to allow the infected material to be cleaned out. That was ok but caused me to stay in hospital one extra day.

I couldn't leave hospital until my temperature was normal, which they were very keen on, and until I had been to the toilet.

All was well enough by the Sunday and I was on my way home, seven days after the operation.

I had enquired about MRSA before going into the hospital and was told that there had been no cases of it in the Urology Department at all. The infection I had was a low-key type and although was a nuisance, it had no lasting effect on me except leaving the scar more visible, which is not a problem for me.

I left hospital on the Sunday and went to my good friends the Woodlands for the coming period.

I walked out of hospital feeling weak but glad to be going home. Karen our daughter in law drove me home in a people carrier type vehicle. I couldn't have got into a saloon car, as I couldn't bend down.

Each day the District Nurse came in to change the dressings. Because of the infection, the wound was open and I was told it had to heal from the bottom up. I couldn't believe how deep it was. Some form of packing made out of seaweed was prodded into the wound on a daily basis and served to counter the infection. We don't always give due consideration to what other people do with their time, particularly Community Nurses who must see some awful sights and bring much comfort to many distressed and sad people.

The healing was delayed but I got there in the end.

I had a catheter inserted for a period of time. This is a tube that is inserted into the bladder through the penis and feeds into a bottle that is strapped to the shin. Urine drains out of its own accord and it has to be emptied quite regularly. This allows the internal healing to occur. When the catheter was removed it took about six weeks to regain full control of the bladder valve. Men are blessed with two bladder valves; this type of operation removes one of them so the one left has to be developed to do the job on its own. This is done with muscle exercises that I had started before the operation in preparation for the aftermath. For a few weeks I was wearing pads, but the leaks that were a trickle eventually became drips and then nothing. It was hay fever season, not a good time to avoid sneezing. This caused the occasional leak but even that became controlled. Thank goodness. In some cases it can take more than a year to get things under control and in rare cases goes on longer than that.

Within eight weeks of the operation I was physically back up to strength. The ongoing mental adjustments have not stopped since.

Erections, or lack of them, were and are an ongoing problem. I was offered all the help I could have asked for, injections, viagra, suppositories for the penis, vacuum pump, all have given varying degrees of success but this has proved to be an ongoing condition that I am continuing to deal with.

The whole event from diagnosis to my life today, has had a profound effect on me. Changes have occurred within me that I could never have envisaged, some losses, many gains.

MY OUTCOME

'no religion is wrong but neither are they swipe cards to get into heaven'
ROGER KENLEY DAWSON

WITH this experience, I had become acutely aware of my body in a way I hadn't before. The vulnerability of this life surged into me in a way I can't explain. I had meningitis when I was eleven and was seriously ill with that but over time recovered. This was different.

As I began to pay more attention to my body, it became clear that even the smallest changes I made were having an effect one way or another. Focussing my mind on my body and monitoring the changes with some intensity awoke a part of me that had not been awake before.

I became aware of how my mind could easily connect and affect my body beyond the everyday usual connections that are made.

You may also start to be aware of yourself more and noticing aspects of your own body language, maybe recognising characteristics that your mother or father had which you hadn't noticed before.

This is how it was for me. Being diagnosed shocked me into an internal questioning mode, which was on a different level to seeking to get rid of the cancer. Through self-analysis, which I am sure everyone goes through on some scale, I began to understand that I was part of a continuum. I may have thought so before but abruptly I fully realised what that meant. For me, it meant I didn't know anything about myself really. I knew what I was capable of doing, things I had learned to do in this life. I knew the way I was with people and how people were with me. I was aware of what

I thought about myself and what I was doing with my life but I didn't really know me, I hadn't really paid proper attention to me before, it was a bewildering time.

I was becoming just another statistic, expendable and on the conveyor belt of life just the same as everyone else. For the first time, the bottom line was the only line.

I began to question my self-belief, something was happening to me that was beginning to evaporate chunks of the person I had been up until then. A different level of understanding was beginning to drift in, which fired my desire to know more about the nuts and bolts of this existence.

Researching the subject of prostate cancer took me to the finer detail of the human body, fascinating stuff but a bit disorientating when you apply it to yourself. After months and months of highly inquisitive study I became interested in energy and what energy actually is. As I became more fascinated, I began experimenting with energy and found that I had become sensitised to energy fields around people and animals.

A few miles from where I live, horse sales are held every month or so. I had been on many occasions just out of general interest or to take the grandchildren when they have been staying with us.

I didn't go for quite a while when I was not well, but at a point sometime into my studying period, I went along and walked through the huge shed that holds about a hundred and twenty or so horses. I began to feel agitated in my stomach area and within about ten minutes, I was looking for a toilet. At the time I didn't think too much of it but the next time I went to the horse sale it happened again. I assumed I must have developed an allergy to horses and dismissed any further thoughts about it.

It was when reading a book about talking to horses months later that I came across a passage about horse sensitivity. The section in the book mentioned horse sales and the way horses felt at these sales, being sensitive creatures they experience emotions more intensely than we do and it dawned on me straight away that I had been feeling the anxiety of the horses; the washing machine feeling in my stomach was the disturbed energy being given out by some of the horses and I was sensitive to it.

I was fired up by this and decided to delve further into states of mind and energy fields.

All of this took me into the realms of energy healing. All of my adult life I have done things like make warts disappear overnight and healed headaches and toothaches for friends and family without even thinking about it. I regarded these, as no more than party tricks thinking anyone could do it if they tried so never really paid attention to it.

As time has gone on I have developed my sensitivity, the breathing relaxation that I described earlier later graduated into meditation. I know for some, these things are for people who have too much time on their hands but I can tell you that if you haven't tried it, don't knock it.

I am now involved with energy healing or spiritual healing, whatever you choose to call it. My belief at this time is that it is all from the same source. What is for sure is that it works.

If you question this type of healing, think again, consciously you may dismiss it but without realising you have participated probably many times in your life.

When someone dear to you is troubled or upset and you place your hand on their back or your arm across their shoulder, why do you do that? What is happening? You may say we are reassuring them, comforting them. Yes we are doing that but what is it about our actions that is reassuring and comforting.

As a purely physical action it means nothing at all until that is, you add the good intention to it. You may have been upset and someone has done that to you, it could have been when you were a child and you grazed your knee: a comforting touch by a loving parent took away the pain. You accepted their intention, which was to comfort you in your time of need.

If a person is troubled and a comforting arm is offered and is pushed away or the perception is that the intention is not pure and from the heart, the person will not be comforted by the action.

So you can see from this that you are familiar with healing energies, maybe on a less powerful level but they have played a part in your life either from you or to you.

I have magnified my ability by intention to a point where I have been privileged to be able to help people. I have seen some astounding happenings and have witnessed transformations in people, although this isn't always the case. Healing sessions do not always produce amazing results instantly, outcomes range from extraordinary to subtle and the time for the change can be immediate or over a few days.

Healing works on many levels from dealing with a health issue or serve to help someone re-evaluate his or her life, afterwards becoming calm or changing direction, even becoming appreciative of what they already have.

It might be a magic formula in many ways but the healer is not the magician.

My understanding of what takes place is the healer is delivering energy to a person, allowing that person to heal him or herself to their highest good. To be more precise the person accepting the healing is rebalancing his or her own energy. It is not up to the healer who gets well and who doesn't. For me, I am just the deliveryman.

There is always a change of some kind but not always a total healing. I have been amazed at results from one-to-one healing sessions as well as results from distant healing sessions.

If you feel the inclination to try this type of healing, don't dismiss it. This message could have been written just to reach you. If you have the notion follow it through, spiritual or energy healing may benefit you more than you can possibly know.

I have joined the National Federation of Spiritual Healers and have met some wonderful people along with a well of good intention, which I believe to be the active driving force behind all healing acts.

I thank you for reading this book. I have intermixed my own experience with that of the many people I have spoken to who are also affected with prostate cancer, whether it is the man with the condition or his family. I give thanks to them all and trust that some of the information included here has been beneficial to you and yours and has helped you to understand more clearly the nuts and bolts of prostate cancer.

Use this to establish a positive outlook for you and your family.

I wish you well with your future whatever that might hold for you.

REFERENCE

'if, as one door closes another slams in your face,
ask yourself, are you in the wrong street'
ROGER KENLEY DAWSON

THE author is a practising healer engaged in one–to–one or distant healing. If anyone would like more information or to contact Roger for any reason please do so in the first instance at *www.reachformefirst.com* or via the publishers giving a contact telephone number.

The following is with regard to the ongoing UK Genetic Prostate Cancer Study which is a research programme being conducted by The Institute of Cancer Research & The Royal Marsden NHS Trust. Please read the information carefully and if you fit the criteria, please help by volunteering to take part. Contact details are in the information.

UK GENETIC PROSTATE CANCER STUDY

Previous research has suggested that if a man has a family history of prostate cancer this will increase his risk of developing this disease. This is a long-term study, which aims to increase our understanding of the genetic predispositions of prostate cancers. The study is aiming to recruit 21,000 patients by the end of 2012 and is being run by Dr Rosalind Eeles at The Institute of Cancer Research.

There are several parts to the study. These are a family history questionnaire, request for a blood sample for research, request to collect your prostate cancer sample for research, request to view your medical records and a questionnaire about lifestyle factors. You may take part in all of them or only parts with which you feel comfortable.

It is hoped that the information gained from this study will help the researchers to

Find out how many families have a strong family history of prostate cancer.
Work out a mans risk of developing prostate cancer if he has a family history
Find out if a mans history of prostate cancer also increases his
risk of developing other cancers.
Identify other faulty genes that can increase a mans risk of developing prostate cancer (we already know about BRCA1 andBRCA2).
Establish a storage bank of blood and tumour samples that may help future research.

In the long term, the results of this study may help to find ways to diagnose prostate cancer early and to prevent prostate cancer in some men

Eligibility for the study

All patients with prostate cancer at the Royal Marsden Hospital are asked whether they would like to take part in this study.

If you are a patient elsewhere you can take part in the study if you:

Are the only person with prostate cancer in your family and were diagnosed at age 60 or under.

OR

Have prostate cancer and also have a brother, father or family member who has been diagnosed with prostate cancer and at least one of you was diagnosed at age 65 or under.

OR

Are one of three or more members of your family with prostate cancer diagnosed at any age.

A family member can be anyone related to you by blood, eg. Son, father, nephew, cousin or grandfather.

If you think you may be eligible for this study, you can refer yourself by contacting Dr Michelle Guy or Lynne O'Brien (the Study Co-ordinators). Their address is the Translational Cancer Genetics Team, Orchard House, The Royal Marsden NHS Trust & Institute of Cancer Research, Downs Road, Sutton, Surrey. SM2 5PT. Telephone:0208 661 3507 or 0208 661 3667.

PSA WATCH.

**Results-in-ten-minutes machine. Contact:
ELEMENTAL HEALTH CARE. Tel: 0844 4120020.**

<u>PSA levels</u> opinions vary slightly but the following gives an acceptable
picture;

    Age 40 2.0 ng/mL
    52 3.0
    60 4.0
    69 5.0
    74 6.0
    80 7.0

pcpcpcpcpcpcpcpcpcpcpcpcpcpcpcpcpcpcpcpc

CONTACTS

Tenovus. 43, The Parade, Cardiff. CF24 3AB
  Helpline 0808 8081010

The Prostate Cancer Charity. 3, Angel Walk,
  Hammersmith, London. W6 9HX.

Orchid, St Bartholemews Hospital, London. EC1A 7BE.

PCASO. Prostate Cancer Network. 58, Kings Hill, Beech,
  Alton, Hants. GU34 4AN. Helpline 0845 6502555

PSA North of England. Mansion House Chambers, 2,
  High St., Stockport. SK1 1EG. Tel; 0845 456 0678.

Bristol Cancer Help Centre. Grove House,
  Cornwallis Grove, Bristol. BS8 4PG. Tel; 0845 123 23 10

Scottish Association of Prostate Cancer Groups.
  SAPCa. Algo Business Centre,
  Glenearn Road, Perth. PH2 0NJ.
  el; 01738 450415.   Nine support groups throughout Scotland.

www.reachformefirst.com
My website which contains more enlightening information and the latest
news with regard to prostate cancer. Personal contact details are there too.

<u>Microwave oven dangers</u>
University of Minnesota. 1991 lawsuit in Oklahoma(Norma Levitt).
Hans Hertel+ Bernard H Blanc v MFEA March 1993, Wattenwil,
Switzerland.

<u>Fluoride</u>
Observer June 12. 2005. National Pure Water Association.
Dr Peter Mansfield 1998. Greenpeace. The Scotsman. The British
Fluoridation Society. The Human Rights Act.
Environmental Working Group, 1435, U. St., N.W. Suite 100 |
Washington D.C. 20009.